THE
10-DAY
GLYCEMIC
DIET

THE
10-DAY
GLYCEMIC
DIET

LOSE AN INCH OFF YOUR WAIST
THE LOW G.I. WAY

AZMINA GOVINDJI

THE 10-DAY GLYCEMIC DIET

Pegasus Books LLC
45 Wall Street, Suite 1021
New York, NY 10005

Copyright © 2007 by Azmina Govindji and Nina Puddefoot

GiP System and Tables copyright © 2007 by Azmina Govindji

First Pegasus Books edition 2008

Library of Congress Cataloging-in-Publication Data is available.

ISBN: 978-1-60598-021-8

10 9 8 7 6 5 4 3 2 1

Printed in the United States of America
Distributed by W. W. Norton & Company, Inc.

Dedicated to...

As a newly wed, my dedication goes to my stepsons, Edward, Adam and Sean. And to their father, Richard, who continues to provide me with daily doses of laughter and playfulness. Also, to the rest of the Neale family for welcoming me into the clan.

And, finally, to my darling mum, who has more belief in me than grains of sand in the desert.

With special love to you all.

Nina

There is one person who has stood by me in almost every venture for nearly 20 years. His strong values of integrity and humility have helped to nurture my professional journey. He's been there when times were rough; he's been there at times of elation, always balanced, always caring. A rock in my life, my husband Shamil is a most precious blessing and I'm absolutely convinced I would not be the person I am today without his guiding hand.

Azmina

Our joint dedication goes to the late Roslyn Elson, Director of the Diabetes Research & Wellness Foundation, for her faith and inspiration in publishing our first joint book through the charity.

CONTENTS

Acknowledgements

There are so many special and dedicated people we would like to thank, people who have inspired us, helped with the manuscript and worked on meticulous data analysis. There are too many to mention, but a handful deserve singling out here.

For assistance with the GiP system, we thank our special teammate, Smita Ganatra RD, Chief Dietitian, Brent Primary Care Trust. Smita, you are always there for us, especially when we can't see the wood for the trees. Thanks for your objective analytical mind. For data analysis, we thank Zahra Rahemtulla BSc Hons RD, Registered Dietitian, Hammersmith Hospital NHS Trust. Zahra, you assisted us when matters were urgent, despite your own time pressures. Thanks for your professionalism.

To the many dietitians, other experts and national organisations who have offered quotes and tips for this book. Your vote of confidence in us and our work is heart warming – thanks for being there for us. Special gratitude also to our Australian friends and colleagues Professor Jennie Brand-Miller, Philippa Sandall and Kaye Foster-Powell RD, who have guided and inspired our GI journey.

We have updated the GiP tables, and we couldn't have done it without the assistance of the manufacturers and retailers who met our timescales and data requirements with great patience. Specifically, our appreciation goes to our dear friend and colleague Professor Jeya Henry of Oxford Brookes University. Jeya, you could move mountains if you had to. Such data cannot be collected without: the GI International Tables, authored by Foster-Powell, Holt and Brand-Miller; McCance and Widdowson's *Composition of Foods*, Jill Davies and John Dickerson's *Nutrient Content of Food Portions* and 'Glycaemic index and glycaemic load values of commercially available products in the United Kingdom', C. Jeya, K. Henry, H.J. Lightowler, C.M. Strik, H. Renton and S. Hails, *British Journal of Nutrition*, December 2005.

For fitness and exercise expertise, we are grateful to Antonia Parsons, Masashi Miyashita, Loughborough University and Wendy Martinson RD.

To Pat Naylor who provided an honest and valuable critique of the menu plans. Pat, you are always there for us when we need you and your attention to detail has helped us to make those crucial refinements. We would like to acknowledge Sue Gilfrin, who says she is constantly 'on a diet', for her practical tips on what dieters really want.

Thanks also to the manufacturers who kindly offered samples of kitchen equipment for the recipe development: Morphy Richards, Tefal and Richardson Sheffield.

We are grateful also to one of our youngest contributors, Kirsty Perry, A-Level student from London, who conducted a consumer survey that helped to design the final menu plans and recipes. Our other young helpers are always there when there's a manuscript to churn out – Azmina's dear and fun-loving children, Shazia aged 13, and Bizhan aged 15, for helping to create quick and easy recipes and for assisting in the organisation of the final book.

And to Shamil Govindji, for his painstaking efforts in supporting us from start to finish. We couldn't have done it without you.

Finally, a huge thanks to the publishing team at Random House, especially Julia Kellaway and Caroline Newbury, for their endless support and enthusiasm.

EXPERT QUOTES & TESTIMONIALS

Experts

GI alone may not be enough, the Gi Plan links glycaemic index to energy intake, a link most likely to lead to weight loss.

Dr Tony Leeds, Senior Lecturer, King's College, University of London

An easy-to-read, practical guide. Recommended to anyone who wants a healthier, more painless way to lose weight and keep it off.

Richard R. Rubin, PhD, CDE, Associate Professor, Medicine and Pediatrics, The Johns Hopkins University School of Medicine

Azmina has energy and drive and writes with infectious enthusiasm. Despite never deviating from what's scientifically supportable she makes the concept of GI straightforward and accessible to all. A diet of the moment which will stand the test of time.

Angela Dowden R.Nutr., Registered Nutritionist and health writer for Daily Mail, Zest, Daily Mirror and Daily Express

For those with diabetes, losing weight and stabilising blood glucose levels may seem an unachievable goal. Evidence has shown that not only can GI offer the opportunity to do exactly that, but with this comes the added benefit of potentially reducing the risk of long-term complications. In their inimitable way and with their excellent communication skills, Azmina and Nina have made that target appear more attainable.

Our aim is to improve understanding and encourage good self-management skills. Az and Nina are able to communicate GI in an easy-to-understand way, encouraging more people to adopt an 'I can do it' approach.

Sarah Bone, Executive Director, Diabetes Research & Wellness Foundation

In this practical book, Azmina Govindji makes it very easy for anyone to kick-start a low-GI diet for healthy weight loss with her quick and easy menus and recipes that you'll want to try time and again.

Professor Jennie Brand-Miller, Professor of Human Nutrition, the University of Sydney, and author of The Low GI Diet

The GI diet is excellent – I'd recommend it as a safe and effective approach to weight loss for anyone who cares about their health but loves their food.

Sue Baic RD, Lecturer in Nutrition, University of Bristol

Feedback from patients in my clinic on low-GI eating has been very encouraging. A shocking revelation to South Asians; a diet complementary to Asian food, with the benefit of permanent weight loss. A diet based on GI and overall balance can help reduce the incidence of heart disease and diabetes in South Asians.

Leena Sankla, Counselling Psychologist, Cardio Wellness

The concept of a low-GI diet has been of significant use with a much wider group of clients than I first anticipated. Not only does it have a positive effect on stabilising blood sugars for those with diabetes and obesity, but it also clearly spills over into helping with the management of symptoms of other conditions, for example, PMT and depression. I have found the low-GI diet a very useful tool in my work with people who are working hard to recover from a severe eating disorder.

Mary McDermott RD, Freelance and Specialist Dietitian (Eating Disorders), Ipswich

I think the GI concept can really help people to understand what satiety is all about. Using the GI of foods as a basis for menu planning (alongside good basic balanced eating of course!) is a very good way to help the body to relearn appropriate appetite cues.

Jennette Higgs RD, Registered Dietitian, Food to Fit

Readers

This is an inspiring, holistic approach to managing your relationship with food. Not only is it rich in information around healthy eating but the authors have done all the hard work for the reader including putting together menu plans, no-fuss recipes and shopping lists! The motivational angle provides the switch that makes the difference in how to make the sustainable and maintainable changes required to successfully achieve your inch-loss goals. The book provides a consistent, real, feel-good, 'I can do it' factor, throughout. Hugely recommended!

Pat Naylor, Art of Intuition

'I am so encouraged by what I have read that I also logged onto the website and found heaps of info. I have tried every diet plan going with the same results (poor). I can't wait to get started. I am so excited about this I am only sorry I never came across the Gi Plan sooner.'

'I'd like to say thank you for giving me another chance to lose this weight I've been carrying around for years. I received your little free book with *Slimming* magazine and it encouraged me to buy your full Gi Plan so I am going to give it a fair trial. I have tried to lose weight before but I've always failed in the end and regained anything I ever lost.'

'I only started to follow the plan on Thursday last and I am amazed to find that I have not actually felt hunger pangs since I began. And having throughout my whole life suffered with severe constipation, I am already finding this is so much improved … Determined to carry on with the Gi Plan.'

'I find it such a practical book with a commonsense approach.'

www.giplan.com site visitors

Media

I'm a firm believer in healthy eating plans, not strict diets – make use of expert research to ensure you strike an eating and exercise balance to suit your lifestyle.

Jo Schulz, Editor, **Commit to Get Fit** *magazine*

So many diets are strict, faddy and just not sustainable in the long term, so Azmina's Gi Plan is a refreshing change. Sensible and easy to follow, it's so varied you'll forget you're on a diet! A nutritionist and registered dietitian, Azmina knows her stuff – and it shows.

Charlotte Haigh, Freelance health writer, **Mirror, Zest,** **New Woman** *and* **Slimming**

Azmina Govindji is an authoritative voice in nutrition, in a world where faddy diets that can put people's health at risk are all too common. Popular among countless celebrities, a low-GI diet allows you to shed pounds but still maintain a healthy intake of carbs, protein and all the essential elements our bodies require that can be neglected in other diets. It's all about a sensible approach to food – give it a go!

Lisa Pollen, Features Editor, **Star** *magazine*

Press Cuttings

A solid and scientific way to keep the pounds off.

Woman, *10th May 2004*

...will help you lose weight without starving yourself or having to give up your favourite foods. Nutritionally sound, scientifically based and completely un-faddy, it's the diet that will get you to the weight you want to be and keep you there – for good.

Daily Mail, *24th May 2004*

Hmm carbs. If they're your favourite food get on the Gi diet... Good foods include peanuts, spaghetti and milk chocolate. And they call it a diet...? Brilliant news!

New Woman, *June 2004*

The book features an easy-to-follow diet that still includes plenty of carbs. But, best of all, it's guaranteed to leave you with a bikini body that you can't wait to show off on the beach.

Closer, *26th June 2004*

...the new kid on the block is the Gi diet, and... it gets a big thumbs up from most health experts...clear, practical guide that includes great recipes, plus advice on beating snack attacks and eating out.

BBC Good Food *magazine, July 2004*

...worthy of attention for anyone wanting sound weight-reducing advice. Azmina's nutritional background and Nina's expertise in NLP make this book an enjoyable read. An impressive list of testimonials by dietitians and doctors – from academia and media – support this interesting book.

British Dietetic Association Dietetic Adviser, July 2004

...not just another faddy way to shed pounds, but a sensible eating plan for life.

Daily Mirror, 15th July 2004

...the healthiest and most efficient way to lose weight... Their diet and fitness plan can help you lose weight without deprivation and without you having to give up your favourite foods...for the first time you will actually be able to enjoy getting slim quickly and healthily.

Daily Mail, 30th August 2004

Not a quick-fix plan, this book also encourages you to learn healthy principles that will help keep the weight from coming back.

Slimmer, Healthier, Fitter, September 2004

Case Studies

'The recipes look mouth-watering and I'm looking forward to some of the more unusual dishes that sound exotic yet quick and easy. I think this diet is simple and sensible and the highlighted easy-menu choices with the ready-made shopping list are just what I need to get started.'

Hannah

'I found the quick recipes really easy to follow and they really do only take as long as they say! I also like the variety of food available – there's always plenty to choose from and it's great that what would usually be considered 'naughty' treats, like rich tea biscuits and chocolate bars are part of the ten days. This is the only diet I've been on that integrates well-being principles and exercises so it works on the whole person and doesn't just focus on getting rid of fat.'

Karina

'I feel great. I don't feel like I'm dieting at all. I just try to choose the right food and don't snack every half an hour like I used to, because I just don't need to. I'm still trying to lose a few more kilos and I'm sure this is the best way to do it. No dieting but just small changes in your lifestyle and eating healthy food which makes you full but not fat.'

Marta

FOREWORD

The reason I have agreed to write this Foreword is firstly because of my respect for the credibility and experience of the authors, and secondly because this book encourages balanced eating in a way that surpasses simply focusing on the glycaemic index. For any diet to be effective, it really needs to encompass a wide range of nutrients and be in line with recommendations for balanced healthy eating. It should also allow a weight loss of around one to two pounds a week rather than a drastic loss in a short period of time. *The 10-Day Gi Diet* encourages foods from all the five main food groups, even allowing you the odd treat of chocolate, alcohol or peanuts. If you take away a favourite food completely, you are going to feel even more deprived. The flexibility within this plan allows you to enjoy all your favourite foods, eat six times a day and still keep to a healthy weight-loss plan.

Losing weight is simply a matter of taking in fewer calories as food compared to those calories you use up in your daily activities. So for a GI diet to work properly, you must watch your calorie intake. Az and Nina have created a system here that automatically helps you to watch your calories whilst keeping to low-GI foods. This, to me, is the crux of their success. Within this, they package healthy eating advice and a host of motivational boosters that come from their tried and tested techniques. You can go out and buy any diet book, but without first addressing your relationship with food, that diet is likely to have a short-lived effect. This book addresses the underlying causes of being overweight and then, by challenging your thinking, you are guided to build a healthier relationship with food. Equipped with this, you are then given practical nutritional and GI advice all backed up with good scientific evidence. There just isn't another book on the market that covers this and offers a unique system that incorporates GI and calories.

My personal interest lies with waist management. In my many years of reading professional journals, my view is that by focusing on reducing your waist measurement to a healthy level, you are more likely to reduce your risk of developing conditions such as heart disease and type 2 diabetes. Az and Nina have also focused here on waist measurement and there is research to suggest that low-GI diets are effective in helping to reduce abdominal fat storage.

But simply reading a book is not going to give you that perfect shape. I encourage you, deep inside yourself, to really take on board the wisdom in these pages. Set aside that weekend of preparation time. If you are prepared with the right foods in your store cupboard and the right mentality to put in the small amount of effort that is needed, you're more likely to succeed. Fill in the sections in the *Practical Tools* at the back, because actively writing down your goals or recording your achievements helps towards achieving lasting success.

And, importantly, support from others, such as friends, family or a group of people, can encourage you to get the results you want – there is good research on this. So, for your continued success, I recommend you consider attending the Gi Plan workshops, which are mentioned under *Further Support & Information*. By attending an inspirational day that helps you to put all these tips into practice and share issues and successes with others, you are more likely to be able to stay on track.

You have picked up this book because you are ready to make a change. That change could last for 10 days or it could last for a lifetime. Your initial motivation may be to just try it out for 10 days, and that is often one of the best ways to tackle anything. Try out these 10 days, choosing from the tempting menu ideas and taking on board the fitness bursts and motivational guidance. My sense is that once you notice the benefits, you will be encouraged to carry on. Indeed, it is the intention of the authors to encourage you to enjoy balanced low-GI eating in the long term. They will guide you through a more relaxed second phase, called the 'Lose-it Phase', after the 10 days and then ease you into the 'Keep-it Phase', which helps you to maintain your new healthier figure.

I wish you the very best of luck. You've come to the right place…

Dr Chris Steele MB, ChB
GP and resident doctor on ITV's *This Morning*

INTRODUCTION

This is your kick start to a new, healthier you. These 10 days will show you how easy and filling Gi Plan eating can be. How you plan, what you cook, how much you have, how you keep yourself on track, how you stay energised throughout the day, and much more, is all done for you in these pages. And the best news is that there is flexibility too. You can select from a variety of inspiring Gi Plan dishes. Tuna (or Egg) Niçoise, Sesame Prawn Toasts, 10-minute Mushroom Stroganoff, Roasted Mediterranean Vegetables, Crispy Tortilla Chips, pizza, alcohol, chocolate and peanuts are all thrown in – need we say more?

There is an old African saying. Feed a man a fish and he eats for a day. Teach a man to fish and he eats for life. This 10-day diet is designed to kick-start a sustainable and maintainable life-changing, healthy eating plan to support you in getting the results that you really want. After the initial 10 days you will be guided on how to add more foods so that you continue to lose weight steadily and safely.

If you are reading this, you have already consciously decided to make changes in your life. Before you go any further, challenge your commitment to making this work so that you achieve the result you really, really want. See Monday's quiz coming up.

If you are a serial dieter and you are wondering if this book is the one, remember that you can lead a horse to water but...! You won't get results from just buying the book. You will need to take appropriate action. Naturally, we have made this fun, compelling and relatively effortless. It's only 10 days of your life, after all. And – who knows? – you're likely to be so delighted with the results that you may make it a permanent life-changing process. No more diets – this is it!

New broom, clean sweep

Old habits die hard or so you may have heard. Not so! Change happens in an instant. It's deciding to make the change that can take longer. In the case of your old food programme, lose it, don't use it! This book will support you in dumping those old bad habits. Your 10-day plan becomes effective immediately and at the end of the plan you'll be congratulating yourself with the first-hand evidence of a healthier, trimmer you. Think of it as a building process. If you want to build a skyscraper, you must start with the foundations. Your eating choices today affect how you will end up tomorrow.

Today's choices become tomorrow's reality.

Preparation – get going, going, gone!

You start where you start – today. Set aside any **Sunday** and **Monday** you like to prepare yourself mentally, physically and practically. We have built in these two inspirational prep days so that you will be compelled to give this a go and succeed. Fail to plan, plan to fail! With this idiot-proof guide to visible inch loss in 10 days, know with certainty that you can only succeed, effortlessly! We have done the hard work – the calculations – for you, so enjoy the process and give yourself permission to become the person of your dreams by sticking to a few, simple, golden steps, daily.

What's different about the 10-day Gi diet?

The tried-and-tested recipes in this book are a tempting range of some of your old favourites as well as some new and exciting flavours. Think of Baked Flat Mushrooms with Melted Camembert, Pan-fried Turkey Breasts with Cajun Spice and Tarragon, Rustic Red Lentil and Basil Soup, Chicken Fajitas and Beefier Burgers. Need we go on?

And if that isn't enough, interspersed throughout these enticing menu plans are inspirational stories, compelling visualisation exercises and willpower boosters that will help ensure visible results.

It's all about balance, not about restricting or avoiding. It's about maintaining a balance of healthy foods, and balancing what you're eating with practical, short bursts of physical activity that you can do at home or at work. And we tip the balance in your favour by throwing in the all-important key – motivational tips that will make the whole thing effortless.

The 10-day Gi diet in a nutshell

❏ Tempting menu plans that are based on GI, calories and portion size.

❏ Over 70 quick-and-easy recipes, most of which can be on the table in less than 20 minutes.

❏ Morning energisers, power-up tips and wellbeing boosters.

❏ Simple, yet effective exercises to help keep you GiP-fit. All you need to do is have two bursts of 10-minute exercise each day.

❏ Hints and tips that make it easy to eat the low-GI way.

❏ Punchy, practical and fun!

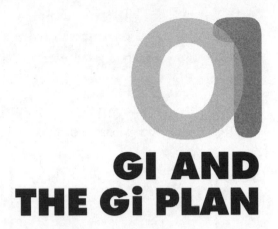

GI AND
THE Gi PLAN

When you eat carbohydrate food (such as bread, rice, potatoes, pasta, cereals and sugary foods), your body breaks it down to glucose (a simple sugar); this can then be used for energy. As the carbohydrate gets digested to glucose, the glucose level in your blood rises. This happens each time you eat a carbohydrate food.

We know different foods cause the blood glucose to rise at different rates. Some carbohydrate foods (carbs) cause a rapid rise in your blood-glucose level; these are best kept to a minimum. Other foods cause a gradual rise in your blood-glucose level; these can help you lose weight.

The Glycaemic Index (GI)

The Glycaemic Index (GI) is a way of ranking foods based on the rate at which they raise blood-glucose levels. Each food is given a number:

❏ Foods that break down quickly are given high numbers – they raise your blood glucose rapidly, and so are said to have a high GI.

❏ Foods that break down slowly are given low numbers – they raise blood glucose more gradually, and have a low GI.

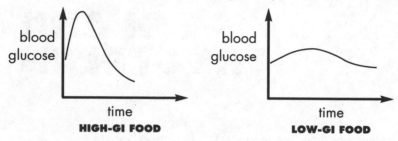

The Glycaemic Index has been researched around the world for years and studies into GI diets have been published extensively, especially in medical journals.

What's so good about GI?

Slowly digested carbs help you feel full for longer, which can delay hunger pangs. It's as simple as that. The tips and menus in this book are based on eating more of these slow-release carbs. Low-GI foods may be more filling because they often have fewer calories, weight for weight, compared with high-GI foods. Many low-GI foods are bulky because of the water and fibre they contain, so they fill you up without piling on the calories. What's also interesting is that when you control your blood-glucose levels, you stimulate your natural appetite suppressants and help maximise fat burning.

There are studies to show that a balanced lower-GI diet can help reduce the fat around your belly. Many diets result in a loss of muscle rather than fat, and since the fat that you store around your waistline is thought to be more harmful than fat stored anywhere else, low-GI diets are particularly healthy.

My GI Tip: There are now at least 10 studies showing that individuals eating low-GI foods lose more body fat than those eating high-GI foods.

JENNIE BRAND-MILLER, PROFESSOR OF HUMAN NUTRITION, UNIVERSITY OF SYDNEY, AND AUTHOR OF *THE LOW GI DIET*

And here's an extra bonus – the effect of a low-GI meal can run into the following meal, which helps keep blood glucose levels even throughout the whole day. This, in turn, helps you feel less hungry.

Choosing foods that raise your blood glucose slowly helps to reduce or even prevent diabetes, obesity and coronary heart disease. Research has shown that people who have an overall low-GI diet have a lower incidence of heart disease. Lower-GI diets have also been associated with improved levels of 'good' cholesterol.

Since foods that take a long time to digest tend to make your blood glucose rise slowly, the key is to include more of these foods in your diet. 'Whole' foods, such as wholegrains, and those high in a particular type of fibre called 'soluble' fibre, such as kidney beans, take longer to be broken down by the body compared with, say, a sugary drink. The grains and beans will thus cause a slower rise in blood glucose. These foods have a relatively low GI. Filling up on low-GI carbohydrate foods at meals and snacks means there's less room for fat (which has double the calories of carbs), so when you're watching your weight, they can also help you keep your calories down.

Healthy low-GI foods – enjoy these

Grainy breads (e.g. multigrain, seeded, granary)
Bran-based breakfast cereals
Porridge and reduced-sugar muesli
Sweet potatoes and new boiled potatoes in their skins
Pasta (choose tomato-based sauces)
Basmati rice
Grains (bulgur wheat, couscous, quinoa)
Nuts (limit to a small handful – 1 oz – a day)
Fruits (fresh, canned in juice or dried)
Vegetables (raw or lightly cooked, fresh, canned or frozen)
Salad (choose low-fat dressings)

High-GI foods – eat less of these

Pies
Sweet pastries
Sugar-rich drinks
Doughnuts
Croissants
Shortbread and sweet biscuits
Mashed potato
Bagels
Baguettes
Sweets
Sugar-rich breakfast cereals

There is extensive research to suggest that a lower-GI diet speeds up the rate of weight loss compared to a standard low-fat diet. Evidence shows that low-GI foods not only help you lose weight, but can specifically help you to reduce the more dangerous fat around your waist.

Weight, waist or body fat?

There are many ways in which you can monitor whether or not you are overweight. You may not even be medically overweight but just feel that, for you, losing a few pounds would be a boost. Doctors and dietitians often use a combination of measures to assess health status. These include measuring body mass index (BMI), waist circumference and/or body fat composition. Here are some snippets on each of these.

Body Mass Index

The body mass index (BMI) is one of the techniques used by doctors and dietitians to assess whether you are a healthy weight. One way to calculate your BMI is to measure your weight (in kilograms) and divide this by your height (in metres) squared:

$$BMI = \frac{Weight\ (kg)}{Height\ (m)^2}$$

A much easier way is to use the chart on page 11, which will help you to work out just how much weight you want to lose to be within a healthy range. Plot your height (without shoes) on the left-hand axis. Plot your weight (without clothes) on the horizontal axis. Make a straight line from each mark and note where the two lines meet. This will show you what your BMI is – your target weight will be in the 'OK' range. Aim for the higher end of this range for now. You may already be within a healthy weight range.

The most desirable range is a BMI of between 18.5 and 24.9. A larger BMI is an indication of being overweight and the higher the figure, the more overweight you are.

However, the BMI is not appropriate for everyone, for instance it isn't suitable for children, young people or older people. Also, if you have well-developed muscles, you may find that your BMI is above 24.9, indicating you are overweight, when in fact you may have a healthy body shape and very little fat.

Low-GI eating is a healthy way to eat, regardless of your weight. Simply allow yourself more GiPs (see *Beyond 10 Days*, page 175) so that you are not losing weight too quickly and make sure you stay within the 'OK' range. It is not safe to aim for the 'underweight' section. And it is more helpful to think of a 'happy weight' rather than a target weight.

As always, if you are concerned about your weight loss or anything else about your diet, you must consult your GP, who may refer you to a dietitian.

Body Mass Index (BMI) Chart

Men and women

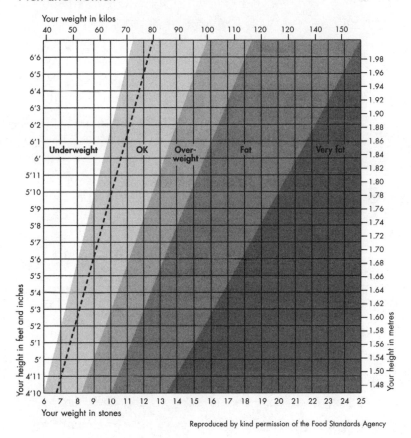

Reproduced by kind permission of the Food Standards Agency

Take the canned beans test

Ever wondered what it would be like to have less weight to carry around? Then have a play at this game. Look at the BMI chart above and find out how many pounds you need to lose in order to get to the upper end of the 'OK' weight range. Now fill a carrier bag with cans of beans or tomatoes equivalent to that amount of weight, bearing in mind that each can weighs about

one pound. Carry this bag around your middle for at least 5 to
10 minutes, walking around while you do so. Not only will this
give you a bit of a fitness routine, it will also help you realise
how much of a strain excess weight can cause.

Now slowly take off a couple of cans at a time and see what a
difference two pounds can make. This is the amount you
could lose in just a week if you follow the 10-Day Gi Diet.

The 'fruit salad' theory

Are you an 'apple-shape' or a 'pear-shape'? This may sound
unimportant, but in fact sound scientific theories have been
formulated using this information. Putting weight on around
the tummy ('central obesity') is said to be associated with
resistance to the hormone insulin, which in turn has been
shown to make you more prone to certain medical conditions.
(Note that a low GI diet can help make you less resistant to
insulin.) You need some body fat to be healthy. It's vital for
basic body functions such as regulating your fertility, body
temperature and appetite and storing energy and vitamins. But
carrying excess body fat, especially around your stomach, could
put you at greater risk of developing heart disease, high blood
pressure and type 2 diabetes.

If you can lower the amount of fat that has settled around
your middle, you are more likely to be able to stabilise your
insulin levels and reduce your risks of these conditions. You
could be within the healthy range in terms of weight and BMI,
yet if you're carrying excess fat around your middle, you could
actually be quite unhealthy.

Here's the low-down. You're in the *watch-out* category if:

☐ You're a man whose waist measures more than 94 cm (37 in).

☐ You're a woman whose waist measures more than 80 cm (32 in).

☐ You're a man of South Asian origin (such men have been found to be even more at risk) whose waist measures more than 90 cm (36 in).

So, getting closer to a pear-shape may actually give you some protection. This is where GiP can help. Choosing foods that are low in GiPs and keeping to the right number of daily GiPs for you, on average, while taking on board our physical activity guidelines (see Chapter 4) can help to reduce excess abdominal fat, getting you into that ideal body shape.

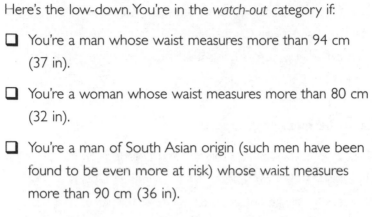

My GI Tip: I'm delighted that this book encourages people to monitor their waist size, when managing their weight. 'Watch your waist' is one of the key evidence-based health messages we promote as part of the British Dietetic Association's annual health awareness campaign, 'Weightwise'.

JILL SCOTT RD, REGISTERED DIETITIAN AND FORMER WEIGHTWISE CO-ORDINATOR, BRITISH DIETETIC ASSOCIATION

The British Dietetic Association recommends that to measure your waist, you first find the bottom of your ribs and the top of your hips. Then measure your waist at a point half way between these two, which for many people is the belly button. Take this measurement now and write it down in the *Practical Tools* section (see Chapter 10). As you keep to the 10-day Gi diet plan, which includes regular physical activity, you will find that both your weight and waist measurements will go down.

Take the measuring tape test

Take a green permanent marker and colour in an old measuring tape from about 24 to 32 inches. This is your target waist range and, if you are within this section, you are considered to have a desirable shape and should not need to lose weight. Now take an orange marker and colour in from 32 to 35 inches. Within this range, you have an increased health risk. If you want to, you can complete the traffic light by colouring in 35 inches upwards with a red marker. The red is often a sign of danger and represents a higher health risk, and it is important that you start to take action.

For men the green band is from 27 to 37 inches, amber from 37 to 40 inches and red 40 inches upwards.

The 10-Day Gi Diet will help you get closer to the amber and green sections of your measuring tape. Measure your waist around the belly button and get motivated to reach your target. Start with getting closer to amber and then, if you can, go for the green.

How much is fat, how much is muscle?

By stepping on the scales, all you know is the number of kilos or stones you weigh. However, that weight is made up of fat, muscle, bone and so on. If you want to monitor your fat loss with your new low-GI eating plan, you can do this more accurately with a Body Fat or Body Composition Monitor, which is a special set of scales you can keep in your bathroom. Obviously, you won't see changes in 10 days, but you will notice a difference as you continue your new healthier lifestyle. And it may also surprise you to see how much (or how little) fat you're actually carrying when you start your plan.

Healthy body fat ranges for adults

AGE	BODY FAT RANGES FOR WOMEN			
20-39				
40-59				
60-79				
AGE	BODY FAT RANGES FOR MEN			
20-39				
40-59				
60-79				

| 0% | 10% | 20% | 30% | 40% |

| UNDERFAT | HEALTHY | OVERFAT | OBESE |

Reproduced with kind permission from Tanita

People within the 'healthy' body fat range have the lowest risk of ill health. 'Overfat' and 'Underfat' carry only a little increased risk. Once people fall into the 'obese' range they are at a very high risk of health problems such as type 2 diabetes, coronary heart disease and certain cancers.

Other benefits of the GI way of eating

☐ Foods that have a low GI are often high in fibre, which can help to reduce the risk of bowel cancer.

❑ Some low-GI foods, such as those high in soluble fibre (beans, peas and lentils), can also help reduce blood cholesterol.

❑ People who are overweight and/or have diabetes are more prone to heart disease. Eating more low- or medium-GI foods as part of a healthy lifestyle can be particularly useful in helping to reduce risks of heart disease in these people.

❑ People who have a condition called reactive hypoglycaemia can incorporate a range of low-GI foods to help stabilise their blood-glucose levels.

❑ The right combination of low- and high-GI foods can help sports performance. Low-GI foods, such as pasta, are great before an important sports event and high-GI foods, such as a glucose drink, provide fast-release carbohydrate, quickly replacing glucose in the blood stream after a sports event.

❑ Low-GI foods are vital when helping to reduce 'insulin resistance' which is the underlying cause of polycystic ovarian syndrome (PCOS).

❑ Low-GI foods can be helpful in combating metabolic syndrome (or insulin resistance syndrome), sometimes called Syndrome X.

What is the 10-Day Gi Diet and how is it different from other GI diets?

The glycaemic index (GI) only tells you how quickly or slowly a food raises blood glucose when it's eaten. But foods with a high GI are not bad foods. Compare potato crisps, which have a medium GI, with a baked potato, which has a high GI. Interestingly, white pitta bread has a lower GI than wholemeal bread – could you ever have guessed that? And some biscuits and cakes have a lower GI than bread. Does this mean we should fill up on these? Of course not!

If you only focus on the GI, then you could be eating foods that are also rich in fat and calories. The uniqueness of the Gi Plan (or GiP) system is that it incorporates a unique set of nutritional criteria. This takes into account not only the GI, but also the energy density (calories weight for weight) and the portion sizes.

> *My GI Tip: All indications at present appear to show positive benefits of lower GI eating. If you look at the health of the nation as a whole, serious consideration has to be given towards formulating food and lifestyle around the Gi Plan.*
> MICHAEL LIVINGSTON, THE DIRECTOR, H•E•A•R•T UK

GI or GL?

GI is a measure of the carbohydrate quality of a food. As you've learnt, GI is a rating that indicates how quickly a carbohydrate food will be broken down into sugar and therefore the speed at which it will cause your blood glucose to rise. This has an influence on insulin levels in your blood. Lower-GI diets tend to result in lower levels of insulin across the day. When you have slow rises and falls in your blood- glucose level, less insulin is required to store this sugar. This helps to regulate your energy levels. Insulin also plays a key role in fat storage and so when you have higher levels of insulin circulating in the body, you are forced to burn carbohydrate instead of fat. But it is the fat that you want to burn off, since burning carbohydrate won't necessarily help you to lose weight. So it is crucial to choose those carbohydrates that give you a slow steady rise in blood sugar, and this is what the Gi diet is all about.

Glycaemic load or GL reflects the quality and quantity of carbohydrate. It is calculated using the GI number as well as the amount of carbohydrate in a particular serving of a food. GL is higher for high GI foods that you might eat in large quantities. Low GL foods can be low in carbohydrate. If there were a scale of the GL value of foods, those that are lowest in carbohydrate are likely to be at the lower end of this scale. So, if you use GL alone, this may not necessarily be a healthy way to eat, as you may be cutting down on carbs and you could be eating a lot of fat and protein while still keeping to a low-GL diet. The key to getting the best blood glucose response is to eat more low-GI carbohydrate foods, not to eat less carbohydrate.

In theory, it's probably best to consider both GI and GL, but this can get very confusing. Using GI with controlled portion size, calories and balanced nutrition offers you the best way of choosing healthy foods as part of your weight loss plan.

The GiP system used in this book helps to reduce the limitations of using either GI or GL on their own. GiP takes into account not only the GI, but also the serving size of a food, including the amount of carbs. And it goes even further. By combining the GI value with calories and serving size, GiP gives you a unique rating that can help you to make healthier lower-GI choices in appropriate amounts for weight loss.

What are GiPs?

The GiP system is really very easy. Food items have been given a score, called a GiP (pronounced 'jip'). Now imagine that you're given a pot of GiPs each day, which you can spend to eat the foods you want. Just as you would spend money to buy food from a shop, here you can choose which foods you spend your GiPs on that day. So you are in control of what you eat.

In the 10-day Gi Diet, all the GiPs have been calculated for you within the menu plans and there is no need for you to do any counting. However, as a general rule after those 10 days, it makes sense to keep as close as you can to your target daily GiPs (more on this in Chapter 6). Each new day you will get another set of GiPs to spend – just like going to the cash machine – but here, the GiPs come to you!

You'll learn how to make your GiPs go further by choosing wisely, so you lose weight without going hungry. What's more, you even get a bonus – you follow some basic tips and you'll end up having a nutritious and balanced diet without thinking too much about it. So you'll not only lose weight, but you'll also be looking after the most important tool in your life – your body.

All this will help you learn new skills and behaviours that will soon become habits that you do almost without thinking, like driving a car or swimming. This soon becomes a lifestyle change and so lasts forever!

The uniqueness of the Gi Plan (or GiP) system is that it incorporates a distinctive set of nutritional criteria. This takes into account not only the GI, but also the energy density (calories, weight for weight) and the portion sizes. Simple and sensible.

What if I'm not interested in counting GiPs?

In that case just ignore all reference to GiPs and you're there. This book is still going to propel you towards healthier low-GI eating. As you flick through these pages, you'll notice a bundle of carefully selected, healthy low-GI foods that taste delicious and help you manage your weight and waistline. All the scientific bits have been done for you so you don't need to worry about counting or calculating. Just munch through the meals and take on the tips and you will be enjoying the Gi Plan lifestyle automatically. And the recipes, although GiP-counted, are quick, easy and delicious ways to enjoy low-GI eating.

GI labelling – it's only part of the story

As you scour the supermarket shelves, you will see that some foods boast a low- or medium-GI label. GI is definitely out there, and manufacturers are trying to make it easier for you to see at a glance which foods are appropriate for lower-GI eating. Remember, however, that it's not just about GI. Fat and protein can also influence the GI, so be careful also to look at the label for all the other things that the food product contains.

The key is to make sure you're eating low-GI carbohydrates, as it is these that are digested slowly and so have important health benefits. Use these low-GI labels as guidance; often it's very valuable information. However, what we've done for you here is to take many of those GI-tested foods and put them through our unique set of nutritional criteria to give them a GiP value. Consequently, foods are rated according to their calorie density and portion size as well as their GI number. This gives you a fuller picture of the value a particular food can have as part of your healthier eating plan.

What really matters is not the fat content of foods per se, but a food's 'energy density' (calories per gram).

JENNIE BRAND-MILLER, PROFESSOR OF HUMAN NUTRITION, UNIVERSITY OF SYDNEY, AND AUTHOR OF THE LOW GI DIET

When making food choices at the supermarket, it's helpful to look at how much of a contribution that food is making to your daily food intake, especially in terms of fat, calories, salt and other things. Below is a table of guideline daily amounts to help you keep on track with healther choices.

Guideline Daily Amounts of Nutrients for Adults

Nutrient	Men	Women
Fat	95g	70g
Saturated fat	30g	20g
Sugar	70g	50g
Salt	7g	5g
Fibre	20g	16g

Some GI-tested manufactured foods, along with their GiP values, are listed in the tables near the back of this book, and many of them have been incorporated into the menu plans. That way, you can include quick-and-easy foods that you simply put into your shopping trolley, take home and enjoy. We have only included those foods that would be favourable within this weight-loss plan. Of course, there may be others that are being tested as we write and others that we are just not aware of.

Low-GI foods can help you to control your appetite by making you feel fuller for longer, with the result that you eat less. There are studies that show that people who eat low-GI meals tend to eat less at subsequent meals.

So do let us know through our website (www.giplan.com) if you know of foods that should qualify for being 'Gipped'. We'll do our best to accommodate these foods in future editions of the Gi Plan series.

The GiP rules

These are crucial as they form the basis of the Gi Plan. They are a simple set of guidelines that, when you put them into action, will transform healthier lifestyle goals into reality.

❑ **GiP Rule 1:** Eat three meals and three snacks every day.

❑ **GiP Rule 2:** Keep as close as you can to your daily GiPs.

❑ **Gip Rule 3:** Have one 'meal carb' at each meal, and 2–3 servings of protein each day.

❑ **GiP Rule 4:** Picture your plate in quarters and fill two quarters with vegetables (v, v), one quarter with protein (p) and one quarter with carbs (c). Here's how you'll remember this: veggie, veggie, protein, carbs.

❑ **GiP Rule 5:** Have at least one low-GiP carb at each meal and always have a snack.

❑ **GiP Rule 6:** Imagine the new you every day – a past photograph will help.

❑ **GiP Rule 7:** Have at least two 10-minute bursts of moderate-intensity physical activity every day.

❑ **GiP Rule 8:** Choose a balanced day by having a variety of foods from the different food groups.

The GiP rules explained

❑ *GiP Rule 1: Eat three meals and three snacks every day.*

GI is based on how foods affect your blood-glucose levels so one of the keys to GiP eating is to eat regular meals and snacks; in fact you're eating six times a day! The menu plans in the 10-day Gi Diet ensure that you are spreading your GiPs out evenly and that on average you spend the same number of GiPs every day for breakfast, lunch, and so on. After the 10 days, when you've become addicted to this healthy lower-GI lifestyle, you will be given advice on how to spread your GiPs throughout the day and make your own menus while you include more daily GiPs (*Beyond 10 Days*, Chapter 6). It's good practice to have your main meal at lunchtime and a lighter meal in the evening, but since many people cook their main meal in the evening, you'll notice these menu plans have exciting dishes for you to look forward to – and they only take about 20 minutes to make.

❑ *GiP Rule 2: Keep as close as you can to your daily GiPs.*

The GiP system is based on a set of nutritional criteria that encompass GI and calories, helping you to lose weight steadily, and with good results. Following the GiP system will give you benefits regardless of whether you have a target number of GiPs or not. However, if you have chosen to follow this diet to help you reach a target weight or get into that new outfit in a couple of weeks' time, then you will stand a better chance of getting the results you want if you keep to the number of GiPs that are suggested.

☐ *GiP Rule 3:* *Have one 'meal carb' at each meal, and 2–3*
   servings of protein each day.

The key here is to focus on the **glycaemic response to carbs**,
not just their GI. You can reduce the GI of a meal by adding fat
or protein, but it is slowly digested carbs that are the healthy
way to improve your blood glucose levels. In this book, you are
encouraged to eat lower-GI carbs at mealtimes – we call them
'meal carbs'. By keeping to GiP Rule 3, you are better able to
get your meals balanced. Choose one 'meal carb' at every
meal. Here are some practical tips which will help you to
choose smart 'meal carbs'.

Bread: Choose grainy, dense breads with whole seeds for your
sandwiches or with your main meal. Good choices include
multigrain, granary, stone ground, rye, 100 per cent
stoneground wholemeal, oatbran, barley and pitta breads.
Some manufacturers have managed to lower the GI of white
bread by adding special ingredients. All these breads will help
you to keep to lower-GI eating.

Potatoes: Most potatoes have a high GI; new potatoes are
slightly lower. Potatoes are a nutritious food, however, so rather
than cutting them out, make sure you include low-GI
carbohydrates with them. So, for example, add baked beans or
a reduced-calorie coleslaw to baked potato. (Note that
mashing potatoes raises their GI as you disrupt their physical
structure in such a way as to make them more quickly
digestible.) Alternatively, why not try sweet potatoes or even
yam or plantain? These have a lower GI and taste delicious,
especially when baked or mashed.

Pasta: A favourite lunchtime salad or as your main meal, most pasta has a low GI. Cook until *al dente* (firm to the bite) and remember, watch what you serve it with! The sumptuous recipes in this book show you fantastic ways to dress up your pasta and still get into your dress... How about *Garlic Spaghetti with Courgette Ribbons* (see recipe, page 258)?

Rice: Choose basmati rice, long-grain or brown rice, rather than high-GI types, such as sticky and jasmine rice. For an alternative to pasta or rice, bulgur wheat (cracked wheat) has an even lower GI and tastes great in salads or as an accompaniment to main meals. Have it simple (*Simple Bulgur Wheat*, see recipe, page 215) or spicy (*Lemony Cod Strips with Spicy Bulgur Wheat*, see recipe, page 248). Or you could try quinoa – an excellent low-GI grain, which cooks just like rice but has more texture.

Beans and Pulses: As well as being fantastic on the GI front, beans and pulses are a great source of protein, iron and fibre. Use them frequently – try stir-fried beans, beany casseroles and soups, or just chuck them into any salad, where they will help to lower the GI of the whole meal. Canned beans are a convenient addition to any meal.

Vegetables and Salad: A must for any GI diet, vegetables form the basis of GiP Rule 4: 'Picture your Plate' (opposite) and are great for lowering the GI of a meal. What's more, they're packed with important vitamins, minerals and antioxidants. Vegetables and salad should always feature in your lunch and main meals. Fresh, frozen and canned all count towards your recommended five-a-day amounts – the more variety and colour, the wider the range of nutrients.

Protein: When it comes to protein, there's no need to go overboard, which is often the advice given in some very low-carbohydrate diets. By keeping to GiP Rule 4, you will automatically include some form of protein and you're likely to have an appropriate amount. When you look at the GiP tables, you may notice that some of the protein foods don't seem to be that high in GiPs. This may make them appear very tempting since you get a large portion for a few GiPs. However, eating too much protein can be unhealthy. Rule 3 ensures that you don't double up on protein portions. So, simply make two to three protein choices per day to help keep your overall diet in balance.

The tables clearly label protein foods as well as the meal carbs. Pulses such as beans, peas, sweetcorn and lentils are a great source of protein and they also offer healthy lower-GI carbs. So, this is one food that you may sometimes choose to have as your protein and at other times as the meal carb. So, for example, if you're having *Spicy Baked Beans* (see recipe, page 222) with a tortilla wrap, the beans will be your protein portion and the tortilla wrap will be your meal carb. If you choose to have some roast chicken with a few tablespoons of sweetcorn and a side salad, then the sweetcorn could count as your meal carb with your chicken as the protein.

❏ **GiP Rule 4:** *Picture your plate in quarters and fill two quarters with vegetables (v, v), one quarter with protein (p) and one quarter with carbs (c). Here's how you'll remember this: veggie, veggie, protein, carbs.*

Imagine you have a couple of chopsticks and you place them across each other on your plate so that the plate is split into four quarters. Two parts are to be filled with the veggies and/or salad, one with the meat, fish, pulses, etc. And the last quarter is for the starchy food such as potatoes, pasta or rice.

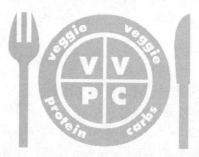

In this way, you will instinctively keep to healthier proportions. Try thinking of meals as 'two veg plus meat', rather than meat and two veg. The vegetables are best treated as an integral part of the meal. Having your plate piled up with veg and salad is a great way to make sure you get a range of vitamins and minerals. You'll also find that most of these foods are either GiP-free or very low in GiPs, so they'll fill you up and keep you trim. For a GiP-free option, you can enjoy most vegetables and salads (choose a fat-free dressing), or you could experiment with the recipes in this book, such as *Roasted Mediterranean Vegetables* (see recipe, page 217) or *Hot and Sour Soup* (see recipe, page 205). Any after dinner fruits count in the veggie section.

If the VVPC plate is the only advice that you take on, you will automatically be enjoying lower-GI eating and this on its own can help you towards your waistline and weight targets.

Remember, slowly digested carbs are those that have health- and weight-loss benefits. So foods such as beans, peas, sweetcorn, chickpeas and lentils, sometimes called 'low-glycaemic carbohydrates', are the ones to reach for. This is why GiP Rule 3 (page 25) clearly encourages you to have one 'meal carb' at each meal. This ensures that you have a low-GI carbohydrate, such as pasta, grainy or seeded breads, bulgur wheat, basmati rice, beans, chickpeas, sweetcorn and so on.

The GiP-free salads and vegetables are your best friends, not only for good health, but also in terms of weight loss, because they are very low in calories. So piling up two of the imaginary quarters on your plate with vegetables and salads makes good sense all round. The only place it doesn't go round is your waist!

The menu plans in the 10-day diet make picturing your plate even easier. You'll notice that many of them actually show you how a particular meal fits into this 'picture your plate' strategy. For example, on day four of your 10-day Gi diet, dinner could look something like this:

Thai-style Trout with Basil and Ginger
Stir-fried Noodles with Crispy Vegetables
Oriental tomato wedges
Fresh pear

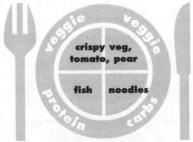

My GI Tip: I love the VVPC Plate tip. I could see how it worked for meat and two veg, but the pictures in these menu plans help me to use VVPC even for a sandwich and fruit.

PAT NAYLOR, ART OF INTUITION

☐ **GiP Rule 5:** Have at least one low-GiP carb at each meal and always have a snack.

This rule is an essential part of the diet. Making sure you have a snack helps to keep your blood-glucose levels steady throughout the day. Healthy snacks help to sustain your energy levels. They may also help keep you alert when you feel you need a nap in the middle of the day. With GI eating, lower-GI snacks can be your ally, as they help to keep your performance and concentration levels at their optimum. What's more, they can positively help you watch that waistline, since a feeling of fullness between meals will mean you're less likely to reach for the biscuit tin or raid the fridge at the earliest moment.

By spreading your intake of starchy food evenly throughout the day and by choosing low-GiP carbs, you're more likely to achieve desirable blood-glucose levels. Here's a simplified way of looking at this:

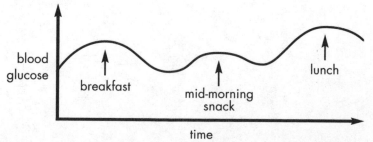

❏ *GiP Rule 6: Imagine the new you every day – a past photograph will help.*

Whatever you focus your attention on, you begin to create as part of your reality. As you imagine yourself at your happy weight, the actions you consequently take will be in line with this image. This means you're more likely to choose the healthier food options rather than acting out of past habits such as filling up on junk foods. We have created our very own DreamBoard™ for you to attach your photograph to. This way, you'll be reminded of it daily and it will spur you on to stick with your outcomes during the 10-day Gi Diet.

❏ *GiP Rule 7: Have at least two 10-minute bursts of moderate-intensity physical activity every day.*

The 10-Day Gi Diet recommends short chunks of regular physical activity that are easy to fit into your daily routine. Being physically active while taking part in any weight loss programme is integral to long-term success. Whatever your age, at least 30 minutes of moderate exercise five times a week is a great insurance policy. It can be as simple as three brisk 10-minute walks each day for five days.

This amounts to 150 minutes in 10-minute slots each week. The 10-Day Gi Diet recommends two 10-minute moderate-intensity bursts each day, which amounts to 140 minutes per week. You can choose how you spend the extra 10-minute burst. You might even choose to do more than 10 minutes – which would be even better! Remember to check

with your GP before starting any activity programme that is
outside your normal routine.

*There is good research to suggest that taking moderate-
intensity physical activity in 10- or 15-minute chunks is
just as effective as 20- or 30-minute sessions.*

❑ *GiP Rule 8: Choose a balanced day by having a variety of
foods from the different food groups.*

Any good diet plan must encourage consumption of an overall
balance of healthy foods. Details of the different food groups
and nutrients can be found in our previous book *The Gi Plan*
or on our website (see *Further Support & Information*, page
367). For now, use these guidelines as a checklist to make sure
you get the balance right:

❑ Keep to the GiP rules on regular eating, lower-GI meal
carbs, protein foods and picturing your plate.

❑ Eat at least five portions of fruit and vegetables every day.
The 'picture your plate' strategy should help you to do this
automatically.

❑ Drink six to eight glasses of fluid (such as water, low-
calorie drinks, herbal tea, milk, tea, coffee) every day.

❑ Make sure you include foods from the five main food
groups (bread, other cereals and potatoes; fruit and
vegetables; lower-fat milk and dairy foods; lean meat, fish
and alternatives such as beans and nuts; and the smallest
amount from fatty and sugary foods).

The 10-Day Gi Diet *is just that – a low-GI plan that is designed for a 10-day period. It is intended as a kick-start. Once you see and feel the results, you will be guided on how to continue your healthier low-GI lifestyle.*

Three GiP tips

❏ **Tip 1:** Under is better than over – choose foods that are under-processed, whole or just cooked rather than overcooked e.g. mushy veg and mash.

❏ **Tip 2:** Most vegetables and fruits have a low-GI rating, and are low in calories and fat – they are your best friends.

❏ **Tip 3:** Nuts are high in calories and rich in the healthier, monounsaturated fat. They are a great low-GI addition to meals, but obviously you don't want to have too many because of the calories they contain. You'll notice that nuts sneak into many of the menu plans. If you're a nut addict, you'll love the *Main Meal Dahl and Peanut Soup* (see recipe, page 259) and the *Nutty Couscous with Lime and Parsley* (see recipe, page 262).

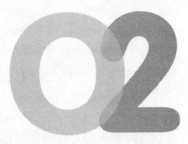

THE 10-DAY
Gi DIET EXPLAINED

The 10-day Gi Diet has been designed to be easy to understand and easy to keep to, with tips, techniques and inspirational thoughts to guide you.

Your Four-step Guide

Each of the 10 days has been neatly organised into four steps. Here goes:

Step 1: Your daily energiser.

Step 2: Select your menu.

Step 3: Get GiP-fit, your two 10-minute bursts of activity for the day.

Step 4: It's time to unwind, congratulate yourself and prepare for tomorrow!

Step 1 – Today's energiser

In this step, you will benefit from a daily energiser that will inspire and motivate you in achieving your 10-day goal. It will support you with what you choose to do and, more importantly, in *how* to do it!

Step 2 – Select your menu

The beauty of these menu plans is that they suit those who just want to be told what to eat, as well as those who like choice. Secondly, if you're someone who likes to count what you're eating and keep to a daily target, then the GiP system helps you to do this in a jiffy. However, if you prefer just to get general information on what to eat and how much, then simply ignore all the GiP values and enjoy the tempting tastes on offer. As we highlighted in the introduction to the Gi plan (*GI and the Gi Plan,* Chapter 1), it helps if you eat relatively more in the daytime and less in the evening. The way this 10-day Gi diet is laid out helps you to do this automatically.

If you like counting your GiPs, read this ...

Research from Dragon Brands in the UK suggests that dieters like counting systems. This helps them to set some sort of target for the day. If you like to count, then you may like to know that these menu plans are based on a total of 17 GiPs per day. Remember, the GiP value is a unique number that refers to the GI and calories in a food. These plans are based on 17 GiPs per day for women (men can have an extra 3 GiPs, making a total of 20 GiPs per day). It is only designed for the first 10 days. After that, you are advised to increase your daily GiP target.

My GI Tip: Although many low-GI foods are generally inherently healthy and are useful additions to the diet, if you are aiming to lose weight then these low-GI foods must form part of a reduced calorie eating plan.

AMANDA JOHNSON RD, REGISTERED DIETITIAN

At the beginning of each day, you will notice how the 17 GiPs have been split throughout the different meals and snacks. Splitting GiPs in this way will help to keep your blood-glucose levels steady, so make sure you don't miss meals or snacks. And you may not realise it, since you are eating all day, but you will be using around 11 GiPs up till lunchtime with only 6 GiPs left for the rest of the day. This automatically means that you will be taking in more of your calories earlier on, giving you the chance to burn them up through your regular daily activities as you go.

After your 10 days, which we call the Start-it Phase, you can increase the number of GiPs you have. You then enter the Lose-it Phase (more on this in *Beyond 10 Days*, Chapter 6). Carry this on till you reach your target weight, and then ease into the Keep-it Phase, a chance to stay slim and trim for ever.

If you simply want menu plans, read this ...

The Gi diet just couldn't be easier. All you need do is decide which of the mouth-watering menus tempt your palate and just go for it. Throughout the 10 days, we guide you through selecting your menu before you start the initial plan and also every evening, so that shopping and planning are much easier.

Obviously, we are not able to provide you with a full shopping list because it all depends on what tickles your fancy as to which menu you're going to choose. However, you will notice a smart shopping section in our 'wicked weekend' (*Getting Ready for Day 1*, Chapter 3) later, and this will give you some pointers before you fill that shopping trolley.

Once you've had this 10-day kick-start, no doubt you will be hooked on the Gi Plan way of eating. You will have learnt the tricks of the trade, such as how to 'split your plate' so you're automatically eating well, you will be able to recognise which foods are likely to offer you a lower GI, and you will have become accustomed to eating little and often with the consequent increased vitality that this offers. All of this will encourage you to keep up your new healthier lifestyle habits. So once you reach that stage, seek some extra pointers from *Beyond 10 Days*, Chapter 6.

What if I don't like what's on today's menu?

Then choose again! There is flexibility within each menu, catering for vegetarians, too. However, if at any stage you feel that today's choice isn't jumping out and saying 'eat me', then all you need do is to choose your own meal from the GiP tables (see page 277). Whether you're a GiP-counter or not, it's easy enough just to substitute the suggested choice with an alternative based on the same number of GiPs as shown. For example, all lunches are based on an average of 5 GiPs. If you don't like the lunch choice and would prefer something else, then look up the tables at the back and make your own 5-GiPs lunch for that day. The same concept applies to breakfast, dinner and the between-meal snacks.

What if sometimes I cook for myself and sometimes for a family?

We've thought of that too! Our survey of dieters showed that this sort of flexibility is important, since not everyone lives alone and not everyone has a family. So what we've done for you is originate recipes that can be adapted to any number of people, so just adapt the quantity of ingredients to suit the number of people you're serving. For ease, most of the recipes serve one, so cooking for two, three or four needs a simple adjustment.

Step 3 – Get GiP-fit

We recommend short chunks of regular physical activity, which is easy to fit into your daily routine. Being physically active while you're on any weight-loss programme is integral to long-term success. If you can maintain some sort of regular activity (and this could be as simple as walking the dog), it can help you keep the weight off once you reach your target. In order for exercise to be of true benefit to you, make sure you see it as a regular habit, like brushing your teeth, and take it as seriously as your driving test.

If you're normally inactive and are now really serious about building up your fitness levels, it's best to **seek advice from**

your doctor. Taking responsibility for your own training schedule is not everyone's cuppa and is perhaps easier for those who are naturally motivated and self-disciplined.

Recruiting a friend or family member to exercise with you – an 'exercise buddy' – can be a great motivator, too. You're much more likely to coax and cheer each other on; turn up even when you'd rather do something else; not let each other off the hook too lightly, and have some great laughs along the way, especially when you choose something that you both really enjoy.

You don't need to exercise for half an hour at a time to get the full benefit – being GiP-fit means doing only two 10-minute bursts of moderately intense physical activity daily. Add this to your current daily routine and you're making a big difference to your fitness and activity levels.

Being active doesn't mean you have to do planned 'exercise' such as an aerobics class or gym session either. If you do, that's great. Remember that just getting off that chair and moving can have an impact. And if you make moving a habit, it will help you to feel less lethargic. Make your 10-minute bursts planned sessions, and aim to feel slightly breathless and warm during your 10 minutes. To check that you're not overdoing it, talk out loud, sing or count up to 10. If talking is difficult you are exercising too hard and should slow down.

GiP Rule 7: Have at least two 10-minute bursts of moderate-intensity physical activity every day.

Step 4 – Time in, time out

Step 4 starts with the opportunity to look back on your day and congratulate yourself on your achievements. No matter how small they may seem to you, they still deserve to get a tick in the box. And here's the fun part. Under the *Practical Tools* section (Chapter 10), you'll notice a chart that tracks your achievements throughout this 10-day plan. This list will grow as the days go by, and you can use them as a great source of motivation on days when you feel you just haven't done as well as you'd like to. It's a chance for you to list every achievement, ranging from refusing a crisp to walking up escalators.

Next, put a few minutes aside each day for your simple but important food preparation for the following day. This includes practical time-saving tips, such as getting your drinks and fruits ready for the next day's lunch or making sure you have the ingredients to hand for your evening meal. Remember, if you invest in a little bit of time the evening before, you'll be much more in charge of what's going on your plate the next day. This will help you to get the results you want. The preparation is an important part of the plan.

Finally, end the day on a calm and peaceful note by setting aside a 'Me Moment'. Each day we will offer you inspirational suggestions, perhaps a short breathing exercise, some thought-provoking questions, or a quiz.

GETTING READY FOR DAY 1
CREATE A WICKED WEEKEND

Sunday – here's what's required

Who's the buddy?

Have a think. Would you like to recruit a buddy to provide extra support and motivation? This person could stay with you all the way through the 10-day programme and even support you with your physical activity. Make a call, share what's involved and what you want to get out of it. Find out what's in it for them so that you can be sure they'll see it through, too. You may be doing them a favour! They too will qualify for Celebration Friday at the end of the 10 days.

What's new?

Decide on a new sport or interest, or choose something that you already love, and commit to doing it regularly as part of the 10-day plan. If you have a chosen buddy, make sure you have a laugh and really motivate each other – especially when one of you wants to flop on the couch! Take silly pictures to capture the memories along the way while you're burning off the calories! Take a few minutes now to consider what floats your boat and write down any ideas that spring to mind.

DreamBoard™

Take some time over the next two days to create your very own personal DreamBoard™. Your DreamBoard™ is a powerful visual tool that reminds you of your goals and what's important to you. When you are clear about what you want, you are more likely to find ways to make that happen. Your DreamBoard™ helps you to maintain clarity and focus. It can be a pin board or a large sheet of paper or cardboard. Use it to attach symbols or pictures that represent the goals that you'd especially like to achieve within the 10-day plan. You can continue to use this well beyond the 10-day plan – and add to it at any time.

Your DreamBoard™ may show any positive image you desire, such as an old photo of you and how you'd like to be, or a cutting from a magazine. You could include colourful pictures of the kinds of delicious foods that you'll be eating, and photos of activities that you'll be enjoying. The list is endless and it's a great 'get started' exercise for your creativity. Make your DreamBoard™ as attractive as you can and place it in a prominent place, so that it acts as a daily reminder. Continue to add pictures, cut out words and/or symbols that represent anything that you'd like in the future. Perhaps include a dream beach holiday?

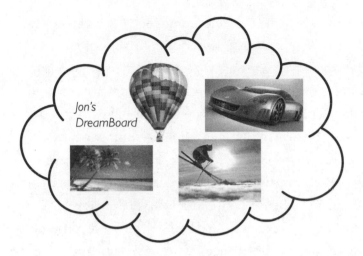

Give some thought to what's important to you regarding your health, wealth, family and relationships, work, interests, hobbies, travel, self-development and your involvement in the community. Capture all of this on your DreamBoard™. For your dreams to become your reality, you must first focus your attention on them, daily!

As you think it, so you become it.

Today's Energiser

Mirror, mirror on the wall... For as long as you see yourself as fat, you will always be fat, even when you are slim! Your self-image is like a barometer, which determines what you focus on and what you think about.

You always get more of what you focus on.

Think of a time when you met someone who was average-looking by your standards, yet radiated an aura of attractiveness, drawing people to them like wasps to a jam jar. Chances are, they think of themselves as attractive, carry their posture accordingly, ooze confidence that others respond to positively, thereby reinforcing their image of themselves as attractive. On the other hand, there are those who have a negative self-image and, as attractive as they are, sabotage any attempts to look their best. Either way, your energy flows where your attention goes and you will get what you expect! Your self-image is determined by who you think yourself to be.

Your behaviour is closely linked to your identity – who you believe yourself to be is how you will be.

Reset your barometer

In the case of many overweight people, despite wanting to be slim, their inner voice says they will remain fat. To break this pattern, the first step is to get used to the idea of being attractive and slim, and focus on what you really **do** want. The mind is automatically programmed to give you more of what you think about, so be careful what you wish for, as you are highly likely to get it!

Your emotions and feelings are influenced by the pictures that you make of the *new* you. These compelling images have an impact on your motivation and energy levels. This shows in your physical body. Perhaps you stand straighter, oozing confidence, shoulders back and sparkling eyes? Your behaviour comes as a result of this process, affecting the food choices that you make. If you think of yourself as a slim, trim, healthy machine, you are far more likely to choose foods that reflect this image of yourself. Your personal DreamBoard™ can help create these strong positive images.

What gets emotionalised gets realised.

When you focus your attention on what it is you really want and on who you really want to become, for example, a slim, healthy, vibrant and energetic kind of person, your unconscious mind will oblige by finding umpteen opportunities to fulfil your goal. Through making use of the most powerful tool you have, you start the process of training your mind, which is inextricably linked to your body, to give you a whole new set of results.

If you always do what you have always done, you will always get what you always got.

A sure-fire way of increasing your chances of getting the results you really want is to **act as if you have already succeeded.** Your mind has difficulty in knowing what's real and what's imagined. Do this exercise to set you up for success for the next 10 days and beyond, and say goodbye to your old self!

Say hello! to the new you

❑ Imagine there is a giant-size television screen right in front of you. Here's where you are going to produce and direct your own unique movie, about YOU!

❑ In this picture, see yourself as the *new* you. Put in as much detail as possible, in colour.

What do you look like? Notice the facial expressions, posture and gestures. What kind of clothes are you wearing? How do you sound? Notice how you speak, listen and laugh. What sorts of things are you engaged in? Perhaps they are activities that you wouldn't have felt comfortable taking part in until now? See how others respond and are drawn to you. Notice how you exude a natural air of confidence and warmth. See the evidence of high levels of energy through making the healthy food choices that a slim, trim, energetic and health-conscious person would make. See yourself getting a regular amount of physical activity that you thoroughly enjoy. How are you doing this?

What else do you notice that makes this *new* you so very compelling?

Feel the inspiration building up in you as you pay more attention to the movie.

❑ Mentally transfer yourself into the picture on the screen and become one with the *new* you image. Make any necessary adjustments in your thinking so that you feel at ease.

❑ In your imagination, think of sometime in the future and imagine this *new* you, going about various enjoyable and stimulating daily events. Ask yourself the questions below and notice how your responses have a positive, feel-good, effect.

What is truly important to me about succeeding with this goal?

How is my life different?

What are the benefits, and how much more can I accomplish in other areas of my life?

What is the positive effect on others?

How much happier do I feel?

Write down the answers, expanding on your initial thoughts. You can use the 'Notes' section in *Practical Tools* (Chapter 10).

Setting your targets

Write down at least three outcomes that you would like to achieve at the end of the 10-day plan and or beyond. Write this down in the *Practical Tools* section, too (page 356). You will need to be specific for this to work really effectively. For example:

- ❏ **I choose to lose half an inch off my waist in 10 days' time.**
- ❏ **I choose to lose one pound at the end of one week.**
- ❏ **I choose to drop a dress size in 4–6 weeks.**

The following exercise will focus your mind, making your results more powerful, attractive and seductive, so that you cannot fail to achieve it!

❑ **Picture** yourself as the *new* you. See the picture in as much detail as possible, as if it has already happened. Remember to include one new behaviour that supports your goal. See yourself hanging around with friends who are supportive and fun. See yourself fitting into that outfit you've always wanted. You too, guys!

❑ **Hear** the comments that others are making to you, congratulating you on your success. What are the great things that you are saying to yourself?

❑ **Feel** the positivity of your achievements and how this enhances your self-image. Soak up the richness that all this brings to your life.

You'll be amazed at the results and just how effortless it is to attract the things that you really want into your life.

Selecting your menu

In Chapter 4 *Your 10-day Plan*, you will see your 10-day plan laid out in front of you. Step 2 asks you to 'select your menu'. With a little planning this weekend, you will be better able to keep to this plan, simply because everything is to hand and you'll make sure you're making the best possible food choices.

Set aside some time for yourself on the Sunday or. Monday before you start to create your 10-day Gi Plan shopping list. Here is how you will do this:

❑ Make sure you've eaten a meal before you do this exercise, so that you are not tempted to reach for something as you read the delicious menu ideas.

❏ Have to hand a pen and some paper for your shopping list and organise your list, if you can, with headings that match the different aisles in your regular supermarket. For example, most supermarkets have the fruit and vegetables section near the entrance, so you may like to make this the first section on your list. Similarly, all the items from the dairy section could be grouped together, as well as those from the freezer compartments, and so on.

❏ Select the menu(s) for as many days as you are happy to do at this stage. For example, you may choose to buy ingredients for the first three days, five days, or week.

❏ Once you've made your choice, simply refer to the recipes (Chapter 8) for the ingredients lists of your choices. The flexibility here is that you can either choose meals just for yourself, or if you are cooking for a family of four, say, simply multiply the quantities and make sure you buy enough ingredients. You may prefer simply to write down the name of the food, rather than worry about precise amounts. For example, rather than writing down '200 ml canned, chopped tomatoes', you might just write 'can of chopped tomatoes' on your list. Take any shortcuts to make it easy for yourself.

❏ If you prefer to have everything laid out for you from A–Z, then turn to page 339 for a shopping list for a selected 'easy-menu' within the 10 day plan. This does not allow you choice during the 10 days, but you never know, the menu that has been selected for this shopping list might just be the one that gets your mouth watering.

We suggest you plan a shopping trip for the Sunday or Monday before you start, and again at the weekend for the next four or five days.

Power tips:

❏ Before you go to bed on Sunday night, make a list of the benefits that the *new* you will bring. Aim for a minimum of 12. Write them down in the *Practical Tools* section (page 352).

❏ Make friends with the body you have in order to get the body you want.

❏ Make a list of all the physical activity and interests that you've ever fancied doing. Commit to trying them all over a period of time. Examples may include: kickboxing, salsa, pilates, yoga, horse riding, skiing. Where appropriate, you can get a DVD to show you how. You can use the blank pages in Chapter 10 for this.

❏ Eating fewer processed foods benefits your waist and your wallet. Get ready to do some simple cooking to get you closer to the *new* you.

> *My GI Tip: Large-scale studies in people with diabetes have found diets that include low-GI carbs are linked to lower waist circumference.*
>
> JENNIE BRAND-MILLER, PROFESSOR OF HUMAN NUTRITION, UNIVERSITY OF SYDNEY, AND AUTHOR OF *THE LOW GI DIET*

Action speaks louder than words!

In a nutshell...

☐ Get yourself a buddy.

☐ List your fun fitness ideas.

☐ Build a DreamBoard™.

☐ Make up your mind to succeed. Failure is not an option!

Monday, Monday

Today's Energiser

How do you rate in this revealing quiz? On a 1–10 scale, score yourself honestly, 10 being the highest.

☐ I am committed to doing what it takes to become the new me. (   )

☐ Today I will set at least three specific goals in relation to my lifestyle change. (Write these down under the *Practical Tools* section, Chapter 10.) (   )

☐ I know I can only succeed. (   )

☐ I know what new choices I need to make to be successful and am committed to making them. (   )

☐ I am clear about the benefits that these changes will bring to my life. (   )

☐ I am clear about how these changes will positively impact on other areas of my life. (   )

❏ I commit to spending up to 20 minutes daily making healthy meals. ( )

❏ With the support of the 10-day Gi Diet, I am ready to make healthy food choices. ( )

❏ I will put time aside daily, for the next 10 days, to follow the simple steps in this book. ( )

❏ I believe that my success is down to me and that it is within my personal control. ( )

How did you score?

Total up your points and then refer to the guide (below).

90–100 Congratulations! Get ready to meet the new you. You are fired up and ready to get going.

70–89 You are so nearly there, mentally. Challenge whatever limiting beliefs you may have. How are these serving you right here and now? Follow the inspirational tips and mental energisers throughout this 10-day plan.

51–69 You need an extra motivational boost. Make a call to a support buddy or someone who would give you extra encouragement over the next few days and follow the power-up tips throughout this book.

If your score is below 50, you haven't committed to making the changes, yet. You are talking the talk but not walking the walk! Give yourself a break while you continue to prepare mentally, and come back when you feel ready. It may help to revisit the 'Say hello! to the new you' exercise, and this time make the images even more attractive. You could even get someone to go through it with you for extra support.

Before you go to bed tonight, commit to setting your alarm 10 minutes early on Tuesday for a motivational booster exercise to get you going first thing!

Shopping the GiP way

As you glance through the delicious menu ideas, you may notice that you already have many of these everyday foods at home. If so, you may have very little adjustment to make. For this new lifestyle to be maintained, it's best to keep to the healthy habits that you currently have and build on them. Making drastic changes to how you eat and live is unlikely to be sustainable. So, as you go through the 10-day plan, make a note of those changes that you found particularly easy, note the food items that you enjoyed eating, so that these can be regular items in your shopping trolley.

Although some of the recipes may call for a particular fresh herb, you can use dried instead. Similarly you can swap any of the vegetables for other GiP-free vegetables in the tables (see page 293). So don't be tied down to absolutely every instruction in the recipe list. Be confident to use your own creativity when it comes to herbs, spices and GiP-free vegetables. The recommendations that are integral to the success of the 10-day plan are: choose lower-GI carbs, cut down on fat, and eat more fruit and vegetables.

If you're someone who just likes to be told what to eat and what to buy, then this section is for you. Flick through your

10 day plan and see if the easy-menu choices (in bold) do it for you. If they do, you're in luck. You will find a shopping list for the easy-menu choices in the *Practical Tools* section (Chapter 10).

If you prefer a pick 'n' mix diet, then start planning for the week ahead. Look through the menu choices and recipes and prepare your list now so that you are ready to set off on Tuesday. Here are some shopping trolley essentials that you will need for most choices:

- ❑ Diet hot chocolate powder

- ❑ Fat-free dressings – choose two or three different types for variety

- ❑ Lower-fat tomato-based pasta sauces (compare labels and choose the lower-fat option)

- ❑ Dried pasta, different shapes, as desired

- ❑ Canned beans and lentils

- ❑ Canned chopped tomatoes and cartons of sieved tomatoes

- ❑ Olive oil spray

- ❑ Roasted peanuts in shells or small packets of peanuts, almonds and/or walnuts

- ❑ Salad vegetables

- ❑ Frozen vegetables

- ❑ Fresh fruit

☐ Dried fruit

☐ Porridge oats, muesli or other low-GI breakfast cereals

☐ Granary, seeded or lower-GI breads

☐ Coarse-grain or regular mustard

☐ Jars of crushed garlic and ginger

☐ Your favourite herbs and spices

☐ Stock cubes, try reduced-salt ones

☐ Olives

☐ New potatoes

☐ Oatcakes

☐ Diet yoghurt

☐ Low-fat natural yoghurt

☐ Other lower-fat dairy products, such as semi- or skimmed milk, or ricotta cheese

☐ Useful utensils, see page 63

Handy recipe shortcuts

Since preparation is the key, here are some hints and tips to help you glide through these 10 days feeling perfectly organised and with everything at your fingertips. They are not essential, but they will be of help.

☐ Buy chicken breast, cut into strips and freeze it in small freezer bags for the 10 days. You can use these in recipes such as *Chicken Fajitas* (see recipe, page 229) and *Chilli Chicken on Granary* (see recipe, page 228).

❑ Boil a large pot of pasta. Let it cool then divide it up in 115 g portions and place in small containers or freezer bags to store frozen and use over the 10 days. This could come in really handy when you want to have dishes such as *Tuna Pasta Salad* (see recipe, page 250) for lunch or *Fettuccine with Creamy Spinach Sauce and Marinated Tomatoes* (see recipe, page 257) for dinner.

❑ Have lots of raw veggies in the fridge so you can make carrot sticks, the Veg Box or the Olive and Cucumber Snack Box (see recipes, page 226). You'll find these ideal for between-meal munchies or for digging into when you come home hungry and need a quick fix.

❑ Give away your party leftovers, and any unhealthy snacks you have lurking in the larder. Out of sight really can be out of mind.

❑ Buy a selection of lower-GI breads, tortilla wraps and pitta bread and freeze them (whole or in batches). You can defrost a couple of slices when preparing the next day's lunch and then have a wrap the following day whilst keeping all the leftover breads fresh.

❑ You don't often see chocolate on a slimming diet, but the 10-Day Gi Diet is more of a balanced lifestyle plan and some chocolate is fine. To prevent you giving in to temptation and eating more than the plan suggests, buy packs of fun-size chocolate and use what you need according to your menu plan. Then freeze the rest so it's out of sight. Defrost as needed next time.

☐ The plan offers a variety of tea-time snacks, such as Rich Tea biscuits, crackers and oatcakes. Store what you need for the 10 days in a tin or plastic container. Put the rest in a separate airtight container for tucking into after your 10 days. You can continue to store, say, a week's supply separately to help keep you trim and avoid over-indulging.

☐ You'll be using delicious mozzarella cheese on one of the days if that's your choice. We advise you to buy a small pack of grated mozzarella, use what you need and freeze the rest to keep it fresh.

☐ Buy handy pre-prepared ingredients such as crushed ginger or garlic – you can get this frozen or in jars.

☐ If a recipe calls for half an onion, be creative and add the rest to a bean salad or choose a dish for the next day that needs onion, such as *10-minute Mushroom Stroganoff* (see recipe, page 261).

☐ Buy dried pulses – such as mung beans and whole lentils. You can either soak these the night before and use them for next day's dinner, or pressure cook them and freeze them in small amounts for the lentil soup and dhal menu choices. Alternatively, stock up on cans of beans and lentils.

☐ If you're tempted by some of the soups, why not make a large pan and either freeze the rest or enjoy it over the next day or so? Some are actually GiP-free (like *Tomato Soup with Crunchy Onions and Green Pepper 'Croutons'*, see

recipe, page 200), so you can actually have as much as you
like at one sitting.

❑ Creatively, some of the menu suggestions use an eat-now-
eat-later strategy. That way, you're only cooking once, as
in making some *Roasted Mediterranean Vegetables* (see
recipe, page 217) for dinner, and you use the leftovers to
mix with ricotta cheese and serve in a tortilla wrap the
next day. It's a great timesaver.

**Be willing to spend 10 minutes preparing the following
day's lunch**

It really makes sense to spend a little time the previous
evening concocting a speedy lunch for the next day. Not only
will this prevent you from picking unhealthy foods that will
make you stray from your goals, but it will also save you time
queuing at the sandwich bar, so leaving you more time for
doing other things such as eating and socialising. And the
bonus is that this will probably work out much cheaper than
buying your usual sandwiches. Step 4 of your 10-day Gi Diet
reminds you to select the next day's lunch and get your
snacks ready.

Being in control of your meals is the best way to ensure you
get results from this 10-day diet. To be committed it really is
worth putting in the planning that is needed. However, there
are times when you just can't put in the preparation time
beforehand. If you feel unable to invest in that time and you go
out to work, then here are some pointers to help you choose
a lower-GI lunch.

Choose this...	Instead of this...
Bread with seeds or whole grains, such as granary, multigrain or seeded bread.	Baguette, white bread, wholemeal bread, hamburger buns, ciabatta.
Bulgur wheat, couscous, quinoa or pasta-based salad, dressed in fat-free (e.g. lime juice) or yoghurt-based dressing.	Salads dressed in mayonnaise or creamy dressings.
Mustard, half-fat soft cheese or reduced-fat hummus as a spread.	Butter, margarine or other full-fat spread.
Extra salad vegetables.	Extra cheese or dressed coleslaw.
Lean meat and poultry without the skin. Examples: three slices ham, lean beef, lamb, or chicken breast.	Fatty bacon, breaded meats such as chicken in breadcrumbs, burgers, full-fat sandwich fillings such as Coronation chicken.
Two tablespoons of grated cheese or two thin slices. Choose, for example, feta (crumbled from a matchbox-sized piece), Edam, ricotta or Camembert.	Cheese and mayonnaise mixtures, large chunks of cheese, full-fat cheeses such as mascarpone.
Two sliced boiled eggs with lots of salad.	Egg mayonnaise.

Choose this...	Instead of this...
Tuna, no mayonnaise, moistened with lemon juice or fat-free dressing. Add sweetcorn, cucumber or peppers as desired.	Tuna mayonnaise.
Beans and peas are a low-GI carb, choose them often. Try kidney beans, chickpeas, sweetcorn, peas or other varieties.	High-GI carbs such as sticky rice. Baked potatoes are a high-GI carb, so when you eat them, match them up with a low-GI carb such as baked beans.
Fresh fruit, dried fruit, diet yoghurt, fat-free fromage frais, reduced-fat drinking yoghurt, reduced-fat hot chocolate, lower-GI cereal or nut bars.	Crisps, chocolate, high-fat, high-sugar snack foods.

Note that if you are not preparing your lunch at home, you will have less control over the number of GiPs you're eating. If you have chosen not to count GiPs, then simply follow the basic guidelines in this book. However, if you prefer to keep track of the number of GiPs you're taking in each day, then simply browse through the food tables (see page 281) to count up the number of GiPs in your choice. Some supermarkets, such as Sainsbury's and Marks & Spencer, have a range of low- and medium-GI sandwiches.

My GI Tip: Make simple food swaps to help achieve low-GI eating. For example, use pearl barley instead of rice in your favourite dishes.
PENNY HUNKING RD, ASD, RPHNUTR. ENERGISE NUTRITION

Useful utensils

There are certain kitchen accessories that make it easier for you to create the recipes or provide convenient ways of taking your prepared lunches or snacks to work. Here is a list of kitchen utensils that you may like to get ready before you start. You may already have most of them.

❑ A standard set of measuring spoons. These can be cheap plastic ones. They'll come in really handy when you're not sure how big a tablespoon is! You can get them from department stores and most supermarkets.

❑ A measuring jug. You will need this when making stock for soups.

❑ A non-stick heavy-based frying pan with a lid. You will find that this will work a treat for omelettes, sautéed vegetables and stir-fries.

❑ A set of kitchen scales. They don't need to be mega-accurate, since you don't need precise quantities (as in baking) for these speedy recipes.

❑ A non-stick pan with lid. This really is an essential item. Non-stick pots and pans enable you to use less oil in cooking, which helps propel you closer to your target.

❑ Time-saving kitchen equipment, such as a pressure cooker, food processor or blender.

❑ Sharp kitchen knives. It's worth investing in at least one quality knife – it does make chopping easier.

❑ Kitchen foil enables fat-free baking and roasting, or use a non-stick roasting tin.

❑ Small containers or freezer bags for freezing.

❑ Handy containers for a packed lunch of sandwiches or salads. You might need one of these for your Olive and Cucumber Snack Box (see recipe, page 226) or Veg Box (see recipe, page 226) which you can tuck into throughout the day.

Tiffin box

Here's your chance to get ready for tomorrow. Invest a few minutes now and you're off to a good start towards waist and weight loss. Decide on whether you're opting for the easy-menu or whether you're more tempted by the other choices. Having already shopped the GiP way for the next few days, you will have all the ingredients and foods to hand.

If you're choosing the boiled eggs tomorrow morning, you might decide to boil them now, store in the fridge, crack the shells and reheat in the microwave tomorrow. Make sure your snacks are handy, either in the fridge or in a bag, ready to take with you if you are not at home tomorrow (or take with you to work). Prepare the delicious smoked salmon sandwich with tabbouleh (should take about 10 minutes) (page 72) or throw the Greek Salad together (page 256).

Take a 'Me Moment'

Try this first thing in the morning, mid morning when you feel you're ready for some time out, and again in the evening. It'll only take moments.

Relax and concentrate on taking long, deep breaths. As you inhale, push your tummy out as if it were an inflatable balloon. As you exhale, draw in the tummy muscles so they collapse inwards. You'll immediately feel a sense of calm enveloping you. Repeat this three times.

Power tips:

☐ Just for fun, buy yourself a pedometer (step counter) and measure the number of steps you take daily. This will encourage you to walk more, dance, pace up and down, or use the stairs. Before you know it, you could clock up 10,000 steps – a five-mile walk!

☐ It takes time to build confidence, a health body and a positive outlook. Be patient with yourself.

☐ Feed yourself with positive self talk. For example, tell yourself: 'I am a healthy, confident, energetic person, I can only succeed in whatever I do.'

☐ Start noticing whether your food is natural or processed. The more chewing it needs, generally the lower its GI. Compare an apple to apple juice, or multigrain bread to wholemeal bread.

It's as easy as 1, 2, 3:

1   Select your menu and create your shopping list (or use the easy-menu choices and shopping list).

2   Measure your weight and waist before or on Day 1 and record this under *Practical Tools* (page 360).

3   Start your 4-step, 10-day plan.

04

YOUR 10-DAY PLAN

All the menu plans in this chapter include an easy-menu
option (highlighted in bold). You will find the shopping list
for the easy-menu options in the *Practical Tools* section
(Chapter 10).

Before you start your 10-day plan, weigh yourself, take your
waist measurement and record your body fat if you have fat-
monitoring scales. Record your results under *Practical Tools*
(page 360).

Remember that even if you're not hungry, the key is to eat the
meals and snacks as shown. This will help keep your blood
sugar and energy levels steady, which is a principle of the plan.
Missing meals will only give you short-term results. And if you
eat all that's on the menu and still feel hungry, go for a GiP-
free snack (see tables, page 281).

DAY 1 (TUESDAY)

Step 1: Today's Energiser

Fire all your motivational boosters to get yourself going with a highly uplifting, fresh and inspirational start to the first day of the new you! Put 10 minutes aside to complete this 'Ring of Success' exercise before starting your day.

❑ Find a quiet spot indoors or out where you won't be disturbed.

❑ Think of what it is like to believe that you can only succeed in whatever you do. Think what it's like to know with certainty that you will be successful in achieving your 10-day goals.

❑ Look ahead a few steps and imagine a 'Ring of Success' in front of you. Make this ring as brightly coloured and attractive as possible. Perhaps there are small lights all around it? Or maybe there is a large spotlight beaming a ray of white light or sunshine into it? When you can see this ring clearly in your imagination, step forward so that you are standing in the imaginary ring, with your feet slightly apart.

❑ Take a few deep, slow breaths, concentrating only on your breath. Now, as you make your breathing even slower and deeper, imagine that on each breath, you are pulling energy up through the soles of your feet. Allow this energy to flow up your legs and torso, into your head and out through the crown of your head. Feel the energy engulfing your whole body, lighting it up inside and out. Repeat this process a couple more times.

❑ As you draw the energy up, allow an intense feeling of success to wash through and over you. Repeat several times, enforcing a sense of certainty around the belief that **you can only succeed.** If it helps, think of a time in your past when you have experienced success.

❑ Find a way to trigger this feeling through a movement, for example, a gesture you may make (like punching the air), or image, or sound (for example, a resounding Yesssss!), or piece of upbeat music. Alternatively, simply press together your thumb and first finger on one hand, or press one of your knuckles, or press an ear lobe. This becomes your personal 'anchor'.

❑ Step out of the ring and then back into it. To ignite the feeling of success, trigger your chosen 'anchor' from above.

❑ Do this a couple more times so that as soon as you trigger the 'anchor', the feeling kicks in immediately.

Fire your secret motivational booster any time you want to recreate the surge of success. You can do this, like turning on a tap, virtually anywhere.

Having got yourself into this **peak state**, you are ready to take on the challenges of the day ahead.

Remember to fire this personal trigger daily, first thing in the morning or during the day, to boost your motivational powers.

Step 2: Select Your Menu (day 1)

Your meal plan is based on a daily target of 17 GiPs, split
on average as follows:

Breakfast:	4 GiPs
Mid-morning booster:	2 GiPs
Lunch:	5 GiPs
Mid-afternoon pick-me-up:	1 GiP
Dinner:	4 GiPs
Evening comforter:	1 GiP

You don't need to count the GiPs; it's all been done for you.

You can make your own menus using the GiP tables so long as
you keep to these amounts.

You can have unlimited amounts of GiP-free veg (see table,
page 293), including as much as you like of the GiP-free
recipes (page 199).

For drinks throughout the day: 200 ml (⅓ pint) skimmed or
semi-skimmed milk, unlimited herbal teas, unsweetened tea
and coffee, sugar-free drinks, water.

For lunch: These suggestions are low GI, filling and varied. You will
be preparing most the previous evening. If some days you can't
be bothered, you can opt for a low- or medium-GI sandwich
from Marks & Spencer's 'Count on Us' range (check labels), a
Sainsbury's GI-tested sandwich (see tables, page 281) or a tailor-
made sandwich from a sandwich bar using our suggested low-GI
ingredients (see *Getting Ready for Day One*, page 43). You are
more likely to get results with the suggested lunches here.

The evening comforter is optional. If you don't like evening snacks, have the comforter at any other time of the day.

Men – have an extra 3 GiPs each day. Check out the tables at the back for GiP values of everyday foods.

Breakfast

Glass of unsweetened fruit juice (150 ml).
1 slice multigrain bread, toasted, with a scraping of half-fat
    unsaturated or low-fat spread.
1 level tsp reduced-sugar jam.
You can swap this for any 4-GiP cereal of your choice (see tables, page 283).
OR
2 boiled eggs.
Fresh or canned tomatoes, if desired.
1 slice granary toast.
Scraping of half-fat unsaturated or low-fat spread.

---

*Quick fix: You could boil the eggs the previous night.
In the morning peel the shell and simply
microwave for a few seconds.*

Mid-morning booster

8 almonds.
OR
1 small pot reduced-fat mousse (up to 100 Kcal, any flavour).
1 fresh apple.

Lunch

Tomato juice (add a dash of Worcester sauce if you like).
Smoked salmon and fresh dill sandwich: 2 slices Burgen soya
and linseed bread, spread with coarse-grain mustard. Fill
with 3 slices of smoked salmon, thickly sliced cucumber,
chopped fresh dill, piles of rocket leaves and cracked
black pepper.

---

*Fat-squeezer: This sandwich uses coarse-grain mustard
instead of butter.*

Wheat-free Tabbouleh (mix together flat-leaf parsley, mint
leaves, 3 diced tomatoes, ¼ chopped red onion. Dress in
1 tbsp lemon juice, flavoured with a pinch of ground
cinnamon, ground all-spice and seasoning).
Fresh grapefruit segments or sugar-free jelly.

---

*If you're a grapefruit lover, choose the grilled grapefruit
option for dessert later on today. That way you can
have half now, half later. And the best news is you
could get your daily vitamin C needs just from this.*

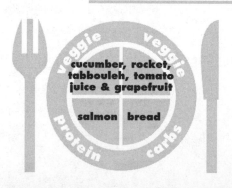

OR

Greek Salad (see recipe, page 256).

I mini pitta bread (ideally wholemeal).

Sugar-free jelly or a handful of strawberries.

Mid-afternoon pick-me-up

I diet yoghurt.

OR

5 ready-to-eat prunes.

Dinner

Fettuccine with Creamy Spinach Sauce and Marinated
    Tomatoes (see recipe, page 257).

Chilli and lime rocket leaves (mix any salad vegetables with
    rocket leaves. Dress in lime juice, paprika, dried herbs and
    chilli sauce.)

I satsuma or I kiwi fruit.

OR

Chicken Fajitas (see recipe, page 229).

GiP-free tossed green salad: simply mix together your favourite
    green salad vegetables such as crispy lettuce, rocket, baby

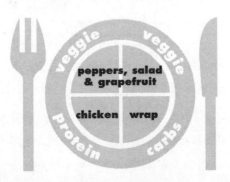

spinach, watercress, celery and cucumber. Throw in some chopped herbs such as flat-leaf parsley or coriander, and flavour with lime or lemon juice. Season to taste.

½ grilled grapefruit: preheat the grill, sprinkle with ground cinnamon and sugar-free granulated sweetener and grill till lightly charred.

If you're not a spice lover, then miss out the spices in the Chicken Fajitas recipe and just season lightly. Still delicious.

Evening comforter (optional)

1 oatcake and a hot drink using milk from allowance.

OR

Olive and Cucumber Snack Box (throw together 10 black or green olives, cucumber sticks, and any combination of the following: celery sticks, radishes, pickled onions, gherkins, water chestnuts).

½ tub of reduced-fat cottage cheese.

Step 3: Get GiP Fit (day 1)

If you're normally inactive and are serious about building up your stamina and fitness levels, it's best to seek advice from your GP. This 10-day plan offers you simple ways of having your two 10-minute fitness bursts as explained in previous chapters.

a) Fitness Burst 1: 10 mins in the morning or at lunchtime
Start today with a brisk walk. Clear the cobwebs and get the oxygen circulating around your brain.

b) Fitness Burst 2: 10 mins at lunchtime or in the evening
Whether it's stairs at your workplace or at home, put 10
minutes aside to walk up and down them.

*You may combine these two bursts of activity into
one 20-minute session if you prefer – the benefits are
the same. But that may put you off at times, so
separating them out may be more sustainable.*

Action point

Improve your posture and flatten that tummy immediately.
Pull in your tummy muscles tightly, stand as tall as you can, with
your shoulders back, chest up and head high. Try it out in the
mirror. Good posture can give you an air of confidence. Do
this daily soon after you wake up or as you're setting off for
work or about to start your daily chores.

*My GI Tip: Do you exercise at lunchtime? Eating a low-GI breakfast
three hours before exercise will increase your body's ability to burn fat
during your exercise session compared with eating a high-GI breakfast.*
Dr Emma Stevenson, University of Nottingham

Step 4: Time in, time out (day 1)

Your two-minute springboard!

Just for a couple of minutes, reflect on your day and notice the positive things that you've done. This could be as simple as walking to the coffee machine rather than asking someone to get a drink for you, or resisting the iced buns in the morning. Every positive action contributes to the new you. Here's your chance to feel elated, not deflated. Turn to the *Practical Tools* section (page 354) and list at least three achievements from today.

Tiffin Box

If you're in control of what you're eating, you're more likely to gain sustainable results. Knowing what's in your lunchbox means you're in charge of what shows on your waistline.

Check out tomorrow's menu plan and select the lunch that you fancy. It will take you probably less than 10 minutes to make the salad, or you may decide to opt for the prepared or bought sandwich option. If you're making the cheese and tomato sandwich, remember to freeze the remaining mozzarella to keep it fresh as you won't be using it again over the 10 days. Throw together the ingredients for the Olive and Cucumber Snack Box (as shown on the menu), so you have this handy if you are choosing it for the mid-afternoon pick-me-up snack. And if you're tempted by the savoury French toast breakfast, you can either make it this evening ready for reheating in the microwave, or just check that you have the ingredients to hand for the morning. It only takes five minutes to make. And if the frozen yoghurt stick gets your mouth watering, pop it in the freezer tonight so it's ready by tomorrow. In fact, you could freeze a few of your favourite diet yoghurts as they are handy for a long-lasting sorbet-type snack or dessert (only 1 GiP). Defrost for about 30 minutes before indulging.

Take a 'Me Moment'

Decide early on in the day how you would like to reward yourself, later tonight, in some small, yet significant way, for getting started! It could be as simple as watching a DVD, enjoying an undisturbed soak in the bath or a swim at the end of a productive day's work.

Sweet dreams…

Power Tips

❑ Congratulate yourself on three things that you successfully achieved throughout the day in connection with this 10-day plan.

❑ You are already making a difference to your body as today you have added low-GI carbs to each meal.

❑ The golden rule today and for the next 10 days (at least), is to climb every mountain! Climbing stairs will tone your legs while giving you an overall body workout.

❑ Move on, think forward and stop beating yourself up over past mistakes. You learn through the stumbling. Tomorrow's another day and that applies to the next 10 days, too!

DAY 2 (WEDNESDAY)

Step 1: Today's Energiser

Start today by spending five minutes to enjoy the Ring of Success exercise from yesterday to get into your motivational **peak state.**

Become crystal clear about why it is important to adopt a healthier lifestyle. It will increase your likelihood of succeeding.

Don't think about ... flying saucers

You will now find that you have to think of flying saucers first, in order to delete the thought! Remember that what you focus your attention on is what you get. This is how the mind is designed. Therefore you are just as likely to get what you don't want! Concentrate on how you want to be; who you want to become; what you want to look like; the healthy food choices that you want to make and the other essential life-style changes that you want to adopt. Ask yourself what simple changes can you make in your current behaviour that will bring the results you want.

The mind doesn't easily recognise a negative command (for example, 'I don't want to be fat!') and acts on the last instruction that you give it (in this case, 'I want to be fat!'). By focusing on being fat, you are reinforcing your negative self-image and your actions will be consistent with this thought. Instead of picking the red, juicy apple, you'll probably revert to the sticky chocolate bun, which will demotivate you minutes later!

Great sports people have found this to be true and instead practise positive thinking. If a tennis player is thinking about hitting the ball into the net, that is exactly where it is likely to go! If the tennis player thinks about hitting an 'ace' — this is what he or she is likely to do.

The same principle applies to dieting. When you direct your focus in a compelling way on what you really do want – a slim, energetic, fit and healthy new you – you are directing your unconscious to prove your success and deliver all possible opportunities to fulfil this outcome. You are the only one responsible for your thoughts and the actions that arise from them.

Repetition, the path to success

Consciously practise positive thinking several times a day until it becomes second nature. Like working out in the gym, repetition is the key to success. You wouldn't expect to get that perfect body by working out once! Similarly, changing your thinking and getting your mind to work on your side to support your goals requires practice too. As you repeat a behaviour, a neural pathway is created in the brain and each repetition strengthens it. Each time you imagine yourself as the healthy, energetic new you, you take another step closer to achieving what you desire. Daily, over the next 10 days, you will be reinforcing the neural pathway of healthy food choices, choosing the foods that will take you nearer to your target. Feel that lightness, confidence and vitality growing with every small step.

Action point

During the hustle and bustle of daily life, if you catch yourself straying, learn and train yourself to catch yourself in the moment. For example, if that extra glass of wine appears to have your name on it, pause and ask yourself how drinking it is taking you nearer to your goal? If it isn't, make another choice there and then, in the moment. Remind yourself of how great it is to wake up fresh and energised in the morning, knowing that you've stuck with your 10-day plan and staved off those extra calories.

Carry this awareness with you today.

Have you ever found you have been thinking about buying something – let's suppose it's this year's must-have handbag – and all of a sudden you see other people with it, or pictures of it pop up everywhere? This is not a coincidence. It's simply a case of what you concentrate on, you create as part of your reality.

Thoughts you dwell on, you bring into existence.

Step 2: Select Your Menu (day 2)

Your meal plan is based on a daily target of 17 GiPs, split on average as follows:

Breakfast:	4 GiPs
Mid-morning booster:	2 GiPs
Lunch:	5 GiPs
Mid-afternoon pick-me-up:	1 GiP
Dinner:	4 GiPs
Evening comforter:	1 GiP

You don't need to count the GiPs; it's all been done for you.

You can make your own menus using the GiP tables so long as you keep to these amounts.

You can have unlimited amounts of GiP-free veg (see table, page 293), including as much as you like of the GiP-free recipes (page 199).

For drinks throughout the day: 200 ml (⅓ pint) skimmed or semi-skimmed milk, unlimited herbal teas, unsweetened tea and coffee, sugar-free drinks, water.

For lunch: These suggestions are low GI, filling and varied. You will be preparing most the previous evening. If some days you can't be bothered, you can opt for a low- or medium-GI sandwich from Marks & Spencer's 'Count on Us' range (check labels), a Sainsbury's GI-tested sandwich (see tables, page 281) or a tailor-made sandwich from a sandwich bar using our suggested low-GI ingredients (see Getting Ready for Day One, page 43). You are more likely to get results with the suggested lunches here.

The evening comforter is optional. If you don't like evening snacks, have the comforter at any other time of the day.

Men – have an extra 3 GiPs each day. Check out the tables at the back for GiP values of everyday foods.

Breakfast

3 triangles of Savoury French Toast (beat 2 eggs and mix in chopped coriander leaves, coarse-grain mustard and seasoning. Soak 2 slices of bread in the egg mixture and fry both sides in 10 sprays of oil. Drizzle on some Worcester sauce. Or see recipe, page 255.)

Eat-now-eat-later 5-minute recipe.

OR

5 tbsp puffed wheat with sliced strawberries and 200 ml (⅓ pint) skimmed or semi-skimmed milk. Add an artificial sweetener if you like.

You can swap this for any 4-GiP cereal of your choice (see tables, page 283).

Mid-morning booster

1 triangle of Savoury French Toast (left over from breakfast). Mug of soup, made up from a sachet.

OR

12 grapes.
1 fresh apple.

Lunch

Tuna (or Egg) Niçoise (see recipe, page 246) with 1 oatcake,
or Sainsbury's Be Good to Yourself Tuna and Cucumber
Sandwich.

GiP-free tossed green salad: mix together your favourite green
salad vegetables such as crispy lettuce, rocket, baby
spinach, watercress, celery and cucumber. Throw in some
chopped herbs such as flat-leaf parsley or coriander and
flavour with lime or lemon juice. Season to taste.

3 plums and 1 firm pear.

OR

**Cheese and tomato sandwich: 2 slices granary or seeded
bread, spread with a scraping of low-fat spread and filled
with 25 g of mozzarella cheese, fresh basil and unlimited
sliced tomato, or Sainsbury's Be Good to Yourself Egg
and Cress Sandwich.**

GiP-free tossed green salad (as above).

Sugar-free jelly.

---

*Buy a small pack of grated mozzarella, use 25 g for this
sandwich, and freeze the rest. That way, it's out of sight
and you have it ready for another day without worrying
about keeping it fresh (you can freeze it for a month).*

Mid-afternoon pick-me-up

Olive and Cucumber Snack Box (throw together 10 black or
green olives, cucumber sticks, and any combination of the

following: celery sticks, radishes, pickled onions, gherkins, water chestnuts).

Tesco Healthy Living Light Strawberry yoghurt (low GI).

OR

1 regular diet yoghurt.

Dinner

Fancy a glass of wine today? Enjoy one glass or half a pint of beer with dinner. Keep strictly to one unit of alcohol.

Citrus Roast Chicken Parcels (see recipe, page 230).

GiP-free Balsamic French beans (add Balsamic vinegar and seasoning to boiled French beans).

GiP-free Roasted Mediterranean Vegetables (see recipe, page 217).

Frozen Yoghurt Stick (see recipe, page 269), made previously.

Try the Coriander Chutney to flavour any meal (see recipe, page 223). The roasted vegetables cook in the oven with the chicken parcels. Both cook in about 15–20 minutes. You can cook vegetables quickly in the microwave if you prefer. Try chopping a courgette and cooking it with button mushrooms, 5 sprays of oil, and herbs and seasoning. It's cooked in about 5 minutes in the microwave.

OR

Red Lentil Dahl with Lime and Coriander (see recipe, page 266).

Serve with 6 tbsp boiled Basmati rice or brown rice (about 45 g raw). You could try Aromatic Basmati Rice (see recipe, page 223).

Mixed Pepper Salsa (mix together ½ red and ½ yellow diced
pepper, ½ chopped red onion and some chopped flat-leaf
parsley. Dress in fresh lime juice and seasoning) or a
simple salad with fat-free dressing.

Strawberry and kiwi kebabs (thread alternate chunks of
1 chopped kiwi fruit and 6 whole strawberries onto
bamboo skewers. Pierce in some whole mint or basil
leaves, if you have them).

*My GI Tip: Remember pulses. They're filling, nutritious,
convenient (canned are fine), versatile, health protecting –
and taste great. When planning or preparing meals, think
how you might be able to slip in some beans or lentils.*
LYNDEL COSTAIN B.SC.RD, REGISTERED DIETITIAN

Evening comforter (optional)

Mug of Marmite or other yeast extract.

Carrot sticks with 75 ml low-fat plain yoghurt for dipping.

*Shortcut: If you can't be bothered to make carrot
sticks at home, you can buy pre-prepared carrot
batons from the supermarket. Yeast extracts are high
in salt, but they are also a great source of B vitamins.*

OR

Diet hot chocolate made up from a sachet with water or
skimmed milk.

Step 3: Get GiP Fit (day 2)

Remember, you may combine these into one 20-minute burst if you prefer.

a) Fitness Burst 1: 10 mins in the morning or at lunchtime
Start the day with a 10-minute jog. Come home full of vitality and energy, jump in the shower and feel great about facing the day ahead.

b) Fitness Burst 2: 10 mins at lunchtime or in the evening
On your bike! Dig out your cycle and get cycling for this 10 minutes. If you haven't got one, borrow one, or buy one second hand, if you don't wish to spend too much.

Listen to your body. You can gain with no pain.
Exercise should be gradual.

Step 4: Time in, time out (day 2)

Your two-minute springboard!

Go to the *Practical Tools* section (page 354) and list your three achievements for today.

Tiffin Box

Choose tomorrow's menu items so you can be prepared: tomorrow's sandwich or wrap will take you around five minutes to prepare. Your fruit, sachet of soup or fruit drinks for between-meal snacks can simply be slipped into your bag in the morning. Check you have all the ingredients for tomorrow's evening meal.

Take a 'Me Moment'

Add another picture or cutting to your DreamBoard™: something that you really want, that may be linked with your 10-day plan.

Power Tips

☐ Simplify your life by increasing your focus.

☐ Regular meals and snacks help keep your blood sugars and energy levels steady throughout the day.

☐ Aim for a 30-minute walk at a pace that makes you slightly out of breath (but still able to talk).

☐ Train the brain to think happy thoughts. Make a list of all the things that bring a smile to your face and practise thinking about them daily. Optimists live longer than pessimists!

DAY 3 (THURSDAY)

Step 1: Today's Energiser

The Feel Great Factor

Circumstances don't reveal a person, they make a person. Make the best of what you already have and let a sense of mental lightness outweigh the challenges when the tough gets rough.

Feel great, here's how…

❑ Eat your meals on a smaller plate to make them look bigger.

❑ Get out at lunchtime so that you can focus your attention on enjoying your food.

❑ Have your evening meal sitting at the dining table and be conscious of what you are eating. Enjoy each mouthful.

❑ Distract yourself at times when you feel a moment of over-indulgence creeping up. Make a phone call, go for a stroll, have a bath, do some housework. Or anything else that floats your boat!

❑ Plan a reward for yourself at the end of the 10 days and look forward to it. Add this to your *Practical Tools* (page 358).

❑ Put your fork down after every mouthful – it will slow down your eating.

❑ Double check you have the recommended low-GI snacks and nibbles close to hand.

❑ Brush your teeth after eating. It helps to take the hunger pangs away.

❑ Frequently revisit your list of 'new-you' benefits. (See *Practical Tools*; page 352.)

❑ Seize every opportunity to nourish your body through exercise. Make it into a game!

❑ Check out your personal DreamBoard™ for a poignant reminder of what's important to you.

Prevention is better than cure

❑ Shop only *after* a meal.

❑ Increase your understanding of your relationship with food by keeping a journal of what you are eating. It will help you to monitor what you eat and make the meaningful changes required to succeed in the future. (See the Mood and Food Diary in the *Practical Tools* section; page 361.)

❑ Halve your eating speed, as if you are doing it in slow motion, and savour every mouthful.

❑ Relieve yourself of the burden of self-obsession by choosing to support a friend or doing some charity work. This is likely to take your mind off food by focusing your time and energy on other issues. You're also likely to feel good by helping someone less fortunate than yourself.

❑ Plan a day to go window shopping for clothes, or anything else that would fit in with the *new* you.

☐ Excess alcohol can be tempting but remember how great it feels to start a new day feeling fresh and alert, knowing you've resisted those extra calories – not to mention that hung-over feeling!

☐ If you do go overboard – enjoy it! Free yourself from the guilt that makes so many people give up. Just get back on track the next day.

Step 2: Select Your Menu (day 3)

Your meal plan is based on a daily target of 17 GiPs, split on average as follows:

Breakfast:	4 GiPs
Mid-morning booster:	2 GiPs
Lunch:	5 GiPs
Mid-afternoon pick-me-up:	1 GiP
Dinner:	4 GiPs
Evening comforter:	1 GiP

You don't need to count the GiPs; it's all been done for you.

You can make your own menus using the GiP tables so long as you keep to these amounts.

You can have unlimited amounts of GiP-free veg (see table, page 293), including as much as you like of the GiP-free recipes (page 199).

For drinks throughout the day: 200 ml (⅓ pint) skimmed or semi-skimmed milk, unlimited herbal teas, unsweetened tea and coffee, sugar-free drinks, water.

For lunch: These suggestions are low GI, filling and varied. You will be preparing most the previous evening. If some days you can't be bothered, you can opt for a low- or medium-GI sandwich from Marks & Spencer's 'Count on Us' range (check labels), a Sainsbury's GI-tested sandwich (see tables, page 281) or a tailor-made sandwich from a sandwich bar using our suggested low-GI ingredients (see *Getting Ready for Day One*, page 43). You are more likely to get results with the suggested lunches here.

The evening comforter is optional. If you don't like evening snacks, have the comforter at any other time of the day.

Men – have an extra 3 GiPs each day. Check out the tables at the back for GiP values of everyday foods.

Breakfast

4 tbsp bran flakes with 200 ml (⅓ pint) skimmed or semi-skimmed milk.
Glass of tomato juice (with a dash of Worcester sauce if you like). *You can swap this for any 4-GiP cereal of your choice (see tables, page 283).*

OR

2 tsp peanut butter and ½ sliced banana on I slice of bread or toast. Put the other half of the banana in the fridge for Sautéed Bananas (page 272) tonight.

No time for breakfast? Settle for some nuts and sultanas (or raisins) on the way to work. Mix 20 g of peanuts (almost a half of a small 50 g pack, or about 2 tbsp) with 1 tbsp of sultanas (they have a lower GI than raisins, but you can have raisins if you prefer).

Mid-morning booster

Mug of lentil soup (canned, bought, dried or home-made).
OR
Tesco Probiotic Original Drink (low GI)
6 ready-to-eat prunes.

Lunch

Ham and mustard sandwich: 2 slices multigrain bread, spread
generously with coarse-grain mustard, 2 slices ham, sliced
beef tomato, piles of watercress.
Sugar-free jelly.

---

*Clever clogs – use coarse-grain mustard instead
of butter. Keep the GiPs low and the taste high.
Or you could use half-fat hummus as a spread.*

OR
Ricotta cheese and spinach wrap: mix together a small tub
of ricotta cheese with ¼ diced red pepper and baby
spinach leaves. Season and pile into a wholemeal or
white tortilla wrap.
3 plums.

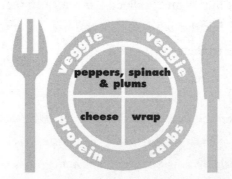

Mid-afternoon pick-me-up

I pear and I apple.

OR

Vie Shot Apple/Carrot/Strawberry.

Dinner

GiP-free Hot and Sour Soup (stir-fry chopped baby leeks in crushed ginger and 10 sprays of oil. Add 450 ml stock, pak choi or baby spinach and chopped coriander. Flavour with Thai fish sauce, wine vinegar, soy sauce and chilli sauce. For full recipe, see page 205.)

Sesame Prawn Toasts (see recipe, page 245).

GiP-free tossed green salad: mix together your favourite green salad vegetables such as crispy lettuce, rocket, baby spinach, watercress, celery and cucumber. Throw in some chopped herbs such as flat-leaf parsley or coriander and flavour with lime or lemon juice. Season to taste.

Fresh orange or Sautéed Bananas (sauté half a sliced banana in 5 sprays of oil. Drizzle with lemon juice and sprinkle sesame seeds on top), using leftover banana from breakfast.

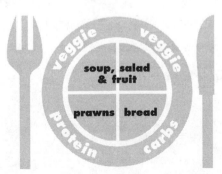

GiP-free means unlimited amounts!
The Hot and Sour Soup cooks in 5 minutes.

OR

10-minute Mushroom Stroganoff (see recipe page 261).

Simple Bulgur Wheat (see recipe, page 215) or Aromatic
Basmati Rice (add a cinnamon stick, 4 whole
peppercorns, 3 cloves and ½ tsp cumin seeds to boiling
water and follow rice pack instructions. Add a pinch of
turmeric if you like it saffron-coloured. Use 45 g of rice
per person).

GiP-free Roasted Mediterranean Vegetables (see page 217),
or salad vegetables in fat-free dressing.

Fresh satsuma, or Sautéed Bananas (see previous page) using
leftover banana from breakfast.

My GI Tip: Good carbs are vital. The greatest mistake that anyone
could make in their daily nutrition is to ignore carbohydrate
and miss out on the health benefits of low-GI foods.
MICHAEL VAN STRATEN, NATUROPATH AND HEALTH EDUCATOR

Evening comforter (optional)

1 rich tea biscuit with a hot drink using milk from allowance.
OR
Diet hot chocolate made up from a sachet with water or
skimmed milk.

Bix tricks: To help you keep to just the number of biscuits on your menu, try making a container with all the biscuits you will need for the 10 days. Keep the others in a separate airtight container and out of sight. You'll need them when you end your 10 days yet still want to keep to low-GI eating.

Step 3: Get GiP Fit (day 3)

Remember, you may combine these into one 20-minute burst if you prefer.

a) Fitness Burst 1: 10 mins in the morning or at lunchtime
Start today by using the stairs to get you going with GiP Fit, day 3. Walk up and down the stairs for 10 minutes. Alternatively, use the bottom step as an 'aerobic stepper'. Simply step up – first with your right foot and then your left – and then step down – right foot first and then left – and repeat, for 10 minutes or as long as you can manage. It's aerobic (and therefore fat burning) and also 'weight bearing', so it strengthens the bones. It's easy and you can listen to music at the same time so it doesn't get boring.

b) Fitness Burst 2: 10 mins at lunchtime or in the evening
Use this time for a brisk walk either during lunch or the evening or whenever you can fit it in. Remember to fit your daily fitness in as effortlessly as possible. This way, you're far more likely to stick with it.

*A good healthy eating plan is complemented by
a safe and effective workout routine.*

Step 4: Time in, time out (day 3)

Your two-minute springboard!

Go to the *Practical Tools* section (page 354) and list your three achievements for today.

Tiffin Box

Choose tomorrow's menu items so you can be prepared.

If you're tempted by the porridge, make sure you have an apple ready too. And if the almond and strawberry yoghurt is more your thing, you could chop the almonds tonight.

If the weather is cold, you might like to make some GiP-free Warming Marrow and Leek Soup (see recipe, page 208) tomorrow. You could make a large pot so that it lasts for more than one serving (remember you can have as much as you like of GiP-free foods). If not, just make sure that you have all the other snacks ready for the following day, especially if you are going out to work.

Select your lunch – if you're tempted by the Spicy Baked Beans (see recipe, page 222), you could spice up the baked beans tonight and put them in a container. Pack a tortilla wrap (separately so it doesn't go soggy) to wrap the beans in. The GiP-free veg box is a trusted friend for those days when you just feel like nibbling. You might want to get into the habit of having GiP-free Veg Boxes (see recipe, page 226) at home, at work and other times for those 'nibbly' occasions.

If you fancy the Tuna Pasta Salad (see recipe, page 250), remember to cook the pasta until *al dente* (firm to the bite), as this helps to preserve the lower-GI value. You can substitute the tuna for a boiled egg or a slice of chicken breast or ham if you prefer.

Remember to have the ingredients ready for tomorrow's evening meal. Freeze your favourite diet yoghurt pot if you fancy a sorbet-type evening comforter. If you prefer a regular frozen yoghurt consistency then pop the pot into the freezer for about 4–5 hours before you need it.

Take a 'Me Moment'

Put a few minutes aside to end today acknowledging all the people and things in your life that make you grateful. Ask yourself the following questions:

- ❑ What am I happy about in my life today? How does that make me feel?
- ❑ What am I proud about?
- ❑ What am I grateful for?
- ❑ Who do I love and who loves me?
- ❑ What am I enjoying most in my life?

Power Tips

❑ When the weather permits, get out into the sunshine, even if it's only for a few minutes and soak up those rays. They'll boost your all-over, feel-good factors while promoting a welcome dose of vitamin D.

❑ Studies show that you burn more fat after low-GI foods.

❑ Save clippings from magazines and papers promoting special offers for an activity you might like to try such as scuba diving or horse riding and give it a go with your chosen buddy.

❑ Pick up a 1 kg bag of sugar to help you feel just how much a little weight loss actually is.

DAY 4 (FRIDAY)

Step 1: Today's Energiser

When you are in a Peak State – that is, feeling every bit as resourceful as you can, on top of things, looking and feeling great and emotionally balanced – you are far more likely to be motivated by your aims and goals in life. This includes your commitment to succeed with your 10-day plan. Here are some great thought-provokers to work through.

Let go and BE!

A good life is a life with a moderate amount of stress only, so that the adrenalin fires you up positively! This way you are more likely to stay happy and healthy and that means the increased likelihood of healthy food choices, too.

When you remove negative language from your vocabulary such as the 'oughts', 'shoulds', 'have tos', 'musts' and so on, you free yourself of the burden of how life 'should' be and how others 'ought' to be!

An attitude of gratitude

Your mind works in such a way that you get more of what you focus on. Acknowledge the things in your life that are already great. In doing so, you are likely to have even more. Your life is already filled with richness, but in the busy-ness of rushing about, you may not always see what's already there.

Stand still for long enough to admire and feel the beauty of what is. Smell the coffee in the stillness of the moment.

Mind and body

You have an intelligent mind and body, which are linked. Whatever happens in one area affects the other. Keeping healthy is to be conscious of nurturing yourself mentally, emotionally, spiritually and physically, in a balanced way. Thinking healthy, happy thoughts will support healthy actions, including your food choices and regular exercise. Physical illness and being at dis-ease with yourself shows symbolically in your body. It's the body speaking in its own language, drawing your attention to what you need to change.

Lighten the load

Laughter is infectious and a great healing tool. Laughter releases happy chemicals that positively affect every part of your being. Imagine the child-like state in you that is ageless, youthful, playful and always grateful to be allowed out. The person who knows how to laugh at themselves will never cease to be amused! When you are having fun, you feel great, work productively and people are attracted to you. Think of it this way: one of your major responsibilities towards others is to enjoy yourself!

 Action point

Spend time with someone you want to be with tonight and hire a comedy DVD. Laugh your little socks off!

Happy days

Happiness is a choice. You can be happy or not, as you wish. It's something you bring into everything you do, say and touch. It's a way of living your life – of being. When you recognise stress, irritation, anger, frustration, remember the rules that govern these feelings live in your head.

Do what you love and learn to love what you do.

A modern tale...

Once upon a time there was a successful and wealthy entrepreneur who rewarded himself by taking a holiday in a small fishing village on a remote island. The entrepreneur asked a young fisherman to take him out for a relaxing day's fishing. The fisherman happily agreed. After a lazy day spent at sea basking in the sunshine, they returned with an awesome catch. Before saying their goodbyes, the wealthy man offered some of his worldly knowledge to the fisherman. He told him that he should increase his prices for the tourists, use the funds to buy better nets so that he could double his catch and expand his fleet of boats.

The young man considered this with interest and then asked, 'What for?' The wealthy man replied, 'Well, that's obvious. You can pay others to do your work while you spend your time fishing and enjoying the sun.'

'Hmmmmm...,' replied the fisherman. 'Now there's a thought!'

Less is more!

And the results don't just affect your health! Often it can be the simplest things in life that bring joy. De-clutter your home and your mind. Examine who in your life drains you when you talk or spend time with them. What in your life has gone past its sell-by date? Make a deal with yourself to tie up loose ends, repay what you owe as early as you can, return what you borrow and only promise what you know you'll deliver! Make a note of these things in the *Practical Tools* section (page 364) under 'De-Clutter'.

Step 2: Select Your Menu (day 4)

Your meal plan is based on a daily target of 17 GiPs, split on average as follows:

Breakfast:	4 GiPs
Mid-morning booster:	2 GiPs
Lunch:	5 GiPs
Mid-afternoon pick-me-up:	1 GiP
Dinner:	4 GiPs
Evening comforter:	1 GiP

You don't need to count the GiPs; it's all been done for you.

You can make your own menus using the GiP tables so long as you keep to these amounts.

You can have unlimited amounts of GiP-free veg (see table, page 293), including as much as you like of the GiP-free recipes (page 199).

For drinks throughout the day: 200 ml (⅓ pint) skimmed or semi-skimmed milk, unlimited herbal teas, unsweetened tea and coffee, sugar-free drinks, water.

For lunch: These suggestions are low GI, filling and varied. You will be preparing most the previous evening. If some days you can't be bothered, you can opt for a low- or medium-GI sandwich from Marks & Spencer's 'Count on Us' range (check labels), a Sainsbury's GI-tested sandwich (see tables, page 281) or a tailor-made sandwich from a sandwich bar using our suggested low-GI ingredients (see *Getting Ready for Day One*, page 43). You are more likely to get results with the suggested lunches here.

The evening comforter is optional. If you don't like evening snacks, have the comforter at any other time of the day.

Men – have an extra 3 GiPs each day. Check out the tables at the back for GiP values of everyday foods.

Breakfast

Speedy Porridge with Grated Apple (see recipe, page 271).
You can swap this for any 4-GiP cereal of your choice (see tables, page 283).
OR
1 almond and strawberry yoghurt: mix together 12 chopped almonds and a strawberry diet yoghurt.

No time for breakfast? Munch through a small banana and four dried dates on your way to work or as you work.

Mid-morning booster

GiP-free Warming Marrow and Leek Soup (see recipe, page
   208), or mug of Minestrone soup, made from a sachet.
1 treat-size (15 g) bar of milk chocolate.

---

*If you can't get treat-size bars, buy a standard bar, cut it into
15 g chunks and freeze in a bag, ideally with greaseproof
paper in between to prevent them sticking together. Then
you just take out a 15 g chunk when you need it.*

OR

1 slice of fruit loaf (no spread).

Lunch

Spicy Baked Beans (see recipe, page 222) in a tortilla wrap or
   Sainsbury's Be Good to Yourself Egg and Cress Sandwich.
GiP-free Veg Box (throw together any combination of the
   following: courgette sticks, cucumber sticks, baby
   gherkins, radishes, cherry tomatoes, celery, baby
   sweetcorn, sugar snap peas, pickled onions, peppers).

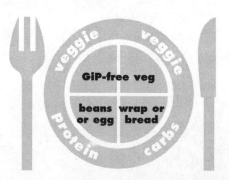

OR

Tuna Pasta Salad (see recipe, page 250).

GiP-free tossed salad, if desired: mixed salad leaves, peppers,
cherry tomatoes and radishes tossed together and dressed
in lemon juice and black pepper or fat-free dressing.

Tesco Healthy Living Light Peach and Apricot yoghurt (Low GI).

Mid-afternoon pick-me-up

2 dates.

OR

2 satsumas.

Dinner

Today's Friday – enjoy a glass of wine or half a pint of beer
with your meal!

Thai-style Trout with Basil and Ginger (see recipe, page 247).

Stir-fried Noodles with Crispy Vegetables (see recipe, page
210).

Oriental tomato wedges: cut 2 or 3 tomatoes into wedges,
throw in a handful of torn basil leaves with a good pinch
of chilli powder, season and add 1 tbsp of fat-free Thai-
style dressing.

1 fresh pear.

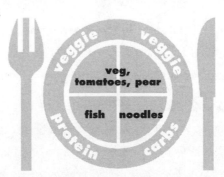

OR

Tomato Soup with Crunchy Onions and Green Pepper
'Croutons' (see recipe, page 200) or other GiP-free soup
of your choice.

Creamy Tagliatelle with Ham (or Chilli Beans) and Field
Mushrooms (see recipe, page 235).

Sugar-free jelly.

Evening comforter (optional)

**Tea with 1 oatcake biscuit (top it with some aubergine pâté
if you like, see recipe for Creamed Aubergine with
Garlic, page 221).**

OR

Frozen diet yoghurt 'sorbet' (simply freeze your favourite diet
yoghurt the previous night or earlier. Defrost about 30
minutes or so before eating).

Step 3: Get GiP Fit (day 4)

Remember, you may combine these into one 20-minute burst
if you prefer.

a) Fitness Burst 1: 10 mins in the morning or at lunchtime
Run for your life! Not quite, but try a 10-minute run if your
fitness level is up to it. If not, substitute with a brisk walk.

b) Fitness Burst 2: 10 mins at lunchtime or in the evening
Dance the night away! If you can, take the time out of your
lunch break, find a few friends or colleagues and an empty
room and go for it. Or, do it in the privacy of your own home.

*A short warm-up followed by a stretch makes the
muscles ready for exercise and reduces the risk of injury.*

Step 4: Time in, time out (day 4)

Your two-minute springboard!

Go to the *Practical Tools* section (page 354) and list your three
achievements for today.

Tiffin Box

Tomorrow's Saturday, yes it's the weekend! If you're not going
out to work, then simply look forward to the scrumptious
breakfast that sets you up for a treat of a weekend.

For lunch, you're going to enjoy Vegetable Pasta in Rich Tomato
and Basil Sauce (see recipe, page 263) or Chilli Chicken on
Granary (see recipe, page 228). If you're at work and these
lunch choices are less practical for you, then simply look up
the tables at the back and create your own 5-GiP lunch, or
glance at the previous day's menus and choose something that
appeals to you.

And just like today, tomorrow evening's meal is accompanied
by a glass of your favourite wine of half a pint of beer.

Take a 'Me Moment'

The quiz – try this to understand more about the difference
that makes the difference!

Q1 *How much of your time is spent feeling stressed, worried and anxious, jealous or angry?*

a) A lot. There is no such thing as stress, only you having stressful thoughts! The meaning that you give to a situation determines your experience. What you are choosing to focus your thoughts on is what causes you to feel the way you do. Choose your thoughts wisely.

b) A few times in a week. When you are in balance and harmony with yourself, your life will feel effortless, like rowing a boat gently down the stream, as opposed to pushing a cart up hill. Some of what you worry about you can't do anything about or hasn't even happened! Some is within your control, so why worry? Take appropriate action instead!

c) Rarely. Congratulations. You are the bodyguard of your own thinking. Your calmness around others will be a great example.

Q2 *How often do you nurture yourself mentally, emotionally, spiritually and physically? (For example, doing yoga, taking a walk or ride in the park, woods, beach or forest, watching a sunrise, smiling and giving compliments and meaning it!)*

a) It's second nature to me. You've mastered the art of a rich and balanced life. Share your learnings with others and become their role model.

b) Not nearly as much as I'd like. Schedule a daily 'me moment' and notice an immediate difference in yourself, your relationships and all that you do. You owe it to yourself.

c) What's a sunrise? Keeping healthy is making a conscious effort to nurture yourself in all the many aspects of your life, to maintain and sustain balance. Practise thinking happy thoughts that will support healthy actions, including your food choices and regular exercise.

Q3 *How much fun, lightness and playfulness do you have?*
a) I've forgotten what it's like. The company you keep will have a major influence on you. Surround yourself with happy and fun-loving people and, like laughter, you too will catch it!
b) A lot. You are already relieving others of the burden of responsibility by knowing how to bring joy into your own life. Continue to take laughter seriously!
c) Only if I remember! Make a pact with yourself to have fun regularly. You'll feel fab, work more effectively and others will be attracted to you like a magnet.

Power Tips

☐ Take laughter seriously! Watch a funny film. The more you laugh the more you release happy chemicals that naturally boost your immune system.

☐ There's research to show that children eating a low-GI breakfast (such as porridge) compared with a high-GI breakfast (such as corn flakes) feel less hungry in class. So low-GI eating could be a healthy family affair.

☐ Music is uplifting. Put on your favourite tracks and become that disco diva (male or female!) Just 20 minutes or more will do the trick.

☐ A lack of sleep is one reason for reaching for sugary snacks. Aim for a good night's sleep, regularly.

DAY 5 (SATURDAY)

Step 1: Today's Energiser

The comfort blanket

Falling back on your personal comfort blanket may bring instant gratification but long-term misery if you reach for solace in food or drink. If your long-term goal is to increase your level of health and fitness, sneaking in those extra glasses of wine may provide a sense of escapism for a while but in the cold light of day, you'll have to live with the consequences of choosing to take comfort in the bottle. This is likely to demotivate you, knowing that you've taken several steps back from where you ideally want to be.

Food and drink cannot feed an emotional hole that may exist in your life. Keeping a food journal will help you identify the emotional need that causes you to give in to the snack attacks or over-indulgence. You may find it useful to write down the cause, such as boredom, stress, sadness, emptiness or some other emotion that is currently challenging for you. Discover who is running your programme – you or your limitations. Once you know what's holding you back, you can begin the changes that will take you in a new direction.

One day at a time will bring you the cumulative long-term achievements that you aim for.

Just as it takes energy to make changes, it costs you energy to remain as you are. There are reasons that keep you where you are: sometimes they are hidden, so you may need to dig deep. These are perceived as 'benefits' as you'll be getting something from them, otherwise you would have made the changes by now.

Whatever the perceived reward is, build it in to your goal so that you can still succeed by achieving the results you want. For example, you may believe, 'People like me as I am.' By becoming more at ease with who you really want to be, you will automatically attract more people to you. Everything about you, your mind and body, will be in harmony, which is often a magnet to others. Carry this belief with you and you'll begin to see immediate results.

Every time you let go of something limiting, you make room for something special in your life.

Action point

Ask yourself, 'What am I prepared to do, that is within my control, for this need to be met in a different and healthy way?' Make a list of several options. Choose the one you feel will really address the issue once and for all.

Step 2: Select Your Menu (day 5)

Your meal plan is based on a daily target of 17 GiPs, split on average as follows:

Breakfast:	4 GiPs
Mid-morning booster:	2 GiPs

Lunch:	5 GiPs
Mid-afternoon pick-me-up:	1 GiP
Dinner:	4 GiPs
Evening comforter:	1 GiP

You don't need to count the GiPs; it's all been done for you.

You can make your own menus using the GiP tables so long as you keep to these amounts.

You can have unlimited amounts of GiP-free veg (see table, page 293), including as much as you like of the GiP-free recipes (page 199).

For drinks throughout the day: 200 ml (⅓ pint) skimmed or semi-skimmed milk, unlimited herbal teas, unsweetened tea and coffee, sugar-free drinks, water.

For lunch: These suggestions are low GI, filling and varied. You will be preparing most the previous evening. If some days you can't be bothered, you can opt for a low- or medium-GI sandwich from Marks & Spencer's 'Count on Us' range (check labels), a Sainsbury's GI-tested sandwich (see tables, page 281) or a tailor-made sandwich from a sandwich bar using our suggested low-GI ingredients (see *Getting Ready for Day One*, page 43). You are more likely to get results with the suggested lunches here.

The evening comforter is optional. If you don't like evening snacks, have the comforter at any other time of the day.

Men – have an extra 3 GiPs each day. Check out the tables at the back for GiP values of everyday foods.

Breakfast

Smoked salmon with avocado and soft cheese: mix 3 slices of
smoked salmon, chopped, with 100g of ricotta cheese,
season and pile into half an avocado. Scatter with a
teaspoon of sesame seeds and serve with firm cherry
tomatoes and lemon wedges.

OR

Cooked breakfast: 1 poached egg, 1 rasher grilled lean
bacon, grilled mushrooms or mushrooms sautéed in
5 sprays of olive oil, chargrilled tomatoes or canned
tomatoes, 1 slice multigrain toast.

Vegetarian choice: substitute the bacon with ½ small can of
baked beans in tomato sauce.

*You can swap this for any 4-GiP cereal of your choice (see tables,
page 283).*

Mid-morning booster

Crunchy apple yoghurt: pot of low-fat natural yoghurt mixed
with a chopped apple.

OR

1 small mango or Mango Smoothie (see recipe, page 269).

*Ever microwaved corn on the cob? Smother a whole cob with 10
sprays of oil, sprinkle with a little salt and add 2–3 tbsp of water.
Cook in the microwave on high for 2–3 minutes (2 GiPs per cob).*

Lunch

Vegetable Pasta in Rich Tomato and Basil Sauce (see recipe,
page 263) or boil 50 g dried pasta and add reduced-fat
tomato-based pasta sauce.

GiP-free steamed lemony courgette ribbons: cut 1 courgette
into long ribbons using a carrot peeler, steam with the
zest of 1 lemon and stir in 2 tbsp of freshly chopped
mint. Season to taste. OR GiP-free Stir-fried Crunchy
Vegetables (see recipe, page 218).

6 slices canned peaches in natural juice, or a satsuma.

*Be label savvy: Compare bought tomato-based pasta
sauces and go for the one with the lowest fat per 100g.*

OR

Chilli Chicken on Granary (see recipe, page 228).

GiP-free Tomato and Mustard Seed Salad (throw together 10
halved cherry tomatoes, 1 tsp coarse-grain mustard, a
handful of chopped parsley and 1–2 tbsp balsamic vinegar
with mixed salad leaves).

1 fun-size Snickers bar.

*Sorting your Snickers snacks: Buy a pack of fun-size
Snickers bars, take out one when it's on your menu
and freeze the rest. This prevents temptation and
you have them handy to defrost as and when
you need them. Or cut a standard bar into
three chunks and freeze them.*

Mid-afternoon pick-me-up

Dip 'n' sticks: 2 tbsp Tzatziki or low-fat natural yoghurt with
celery and pepper sticks.

5 pickled onions (optional).

OR

Oatcake with warmed creamy aubergine: I oatcake topped
with a generous portion of Creamed Aubergine with
Garlic (see recipe, page 221).
Mixed salad vegetables tossed in I tbsp of fat-free dressing.

Creamed Aubergine with Garlic is surprisingly versatile.
Why not make it from a large aubergine and keep
the rest in the fridge. You could have it as an
accompaniment to tomorrow's meal, or a simple
between-meal GiP-free snack another time.

Dinner

**Today's Saturday – enjoy a glass of wine or half a pint of beer
with your meal.**

Chilli Con Carne (see recipe, page 238).
GiP-free *al dente* asparagus tips: steam asparagus tips with a
little crushed garlic till lightly cooked. Season lightly. Or any
GiP-free vegetables of your choice (see tables, page 293).
Tossed salad of your choice with fat-free dressing.
Sugar-free jelly, if desired.

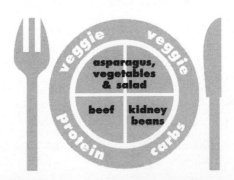

My GI Tip: Lentil and Bulgur Salad is a delicious filling combination of low-GI foods. Cook the bulgur and lentils as directed. Allow to cool. Mix with fresh salad vegetables, herbs and balsamic vinegar and a little olive oil. Delicious.

Sue Baic RD, Registered Dietitian and lecturer in Nutrition, University of Bristol

OR

GiP-free soup of your choice (see list, page 196).

Nutty Couscous with Lime and Parsley (see recipe, page 262).

Mixed salad vegetables tossed in fat-free dressing.

Speedy Salsa Sauce (sauté ½ chopped onion, ¼ diced red pepper and ½ tsp crushed garlic in 5 sprays of oil. Add ⅓ can of chopped tomatoes and a pinch of red chilli powder and simmer for 3–5 minutes).

Sugar-free jelly, if desired.

Evening comforter (optional)

Diet hot chocolate made up from a sachet with water or skimmed milk.

OR

½ large can fruit cocktail, in juice, or 1 fresh apple and 1 firm pear.

Fancy a night-time hot snack? Try stir-fried baby corn: heat 10 sprays of oil in a non-stick pan and throw in some baby sweetcorn. Flavour with soy sauce, black pepper, dried herbs and a dash of lemon juice.

Step 3: Get GiP Fit (day 5)

Remember, you may combine these into one 20-minute burst if you prefer.

a) Fitness Burst 1: 10 mins in the morning or at lunchtime
Enjoy cycling today, either for 10 minutes or for the full 20-minute burst.

b) Fitness Burst 2: 10 mins at lunchtime or in the evening
How about a 10- or 20-minute swim? Swimming is one of the best all-round exercises.

*Toned muscles help to strengthen the body
and burn fat more efficiently.*

Step 4: Time in, time out (day 5)

Your two-minute springboard!

Go to the *Practical Tools* section (page 354) and list your three achievements for today.

Tiffin Box

Tomorrow's Sunday. You're either going to be getting stuck into a roast dinner or enjoying a taste of Italy with Spinach and Ricotta Cannelloni (see recipe, page 264). Either way, it's likely to be a gastronomic experience. No need to do any prep tonight, there will be lots of time tomorrow. You may just want to check you have all the ingredients to hand in case you fancy getting the shopping out of the way tonight.

Take a 'Me Moment'

Exercise daily. Keep mentally alert through practising positive thinking and visualisation. For example, see yourself exactly as you'd like to be and act as if it were already a done deal. Eat a varied range of healthy low-GI recipes and snacks. Get into the habit of practising the VVPC plate strategy, do it often and it will become second nature. There are some blank 'plates' under *Practical Tools* so that you can practise. Physical repetition and mental conditioning, as every athlete knows, are the key to success. They also make the difference between a good athlete and a gold medal winner!

Power Tips

☐ Be spontaneous. Practise curiosity, acceptance, trust, determination and imagination. Watch kids! As you nourish yourself emotionally, you are likely to heal any emotional hole that often gets fed with food.

☐ Try porridge for a change. It's become a quick, convenient microwaveable breakfast, great for cold winter mornings. You may also like to try it as an evening comforting snack.

☐ Keep moving! There is happiness and fulfilment in activity. Use it and stay in service. It's part of the art of living.

☐ Your life has endless possibilities. Write down another three things that will benefit you at the end of the 10-day plan and promise yourself to act on them. Note these in your *Practical Tools* under 'New You Benefits' (page 352).

DAY 6 (SUNDAY)

Step 1: Today's Energiser

What if you were to be more mindful of your feelings of hunger and relate them to an imaginary scale of 1 to 5? Perhaps it would look something like this?

1 – Starving
2 – Pretty hungry
3 – Satisfied
4 – Full
5 – Pigged out!

With the Gi Plan, the great news is that you should never feel ravenous, as the diet is designed to keep you full for longer periods. When you do begin to feel early hunger pangs, it'll be time for your next snack or meal. Often, the brain confuses the first signs of hunger with thirst. Before you are tempted to dive into a snack, try drinking a glass of water to test the signs. Paying attention to your body and the signals it sends to the brain will help you improve your relationship with food, long term.

The secret is to enjoy every mouthful, chew your food slowly and put your cutlery down in between mouthfuls. The other golden rule is to STOP when you are full. It's easy to get sucked into old beliefs that may have been imposed on you during childhood, such as not leaving anything on your plate. Ask yourself, 'How hungry am I feeling right now?' Think back to your scale and know from the answer to leave something on your plate when you have scored a 4 for FULL! This is especially important beyond the initial 10-day plan, in order to maintain your good efforts.

> *My GI Tip: I always give my weight management clients information on portion control and GI. Eating lower-GI foods helps control their appetite, maintain their energy levels and can boost their metabolic rate.*
>
> WENDY MARTINSON RD, ACCREDITED SPORTS DIETITIAN

Step 2: Select Your Menu (day 6)

Your meal plan is based on a daily target of 17 GiPs, split on average as follows:

Breakfast:	4 GiPs
Mid-morning booster:	2 GiPs
Lunch:	5 GiPs
Mid-afternoon pick-me-up:	1 GiP
Dinner:	4 GiPs
Evening comforter:	1 GiP

You don't need to count the GiPs; it's all been done for you.

You can make your own menus using the GiP tables so long as you keep to these amounts.

You can have unlimited amounts of GiP-free veg (see table, page 293), including as much as you like of the GiP-free recipes (page 199).

For drinks throughout the day: 200 ml (⅓ pint) skimmed or semi-skimmed milk, unlimited herbal teas, unsweetened tea and coffee, sugar-free drinks, water.

For lunch: These suggestions are low GI, filling and varied. You will be preparing most the previous evening. If some days you can't be bothered, you can opt for a low- or medium-GI sandwich from Marks & Spencer's 'Count on Us' range (check labels), a Sainsbury's GI-tested sandwich (see tables, page 281) or a tailor-made sandwich from a sandwich bar using our suggested low-GI ingredients (see *Getting Ready for Day One*, page 43). You are more likely to get results with the suggested lunches here.

The evening comforter is optional. If you don't like evening snacks, have the comforter at any other time of the day.

Men – have an extra 3 GiPs each day. Check out the tables at the back for GiP values of everyday foods.

Breakfast

Banana and melon cocktail: 1 under-ripe banana, sliced, mixed with ½ cantaloupe melon, chopped. Serve chilled. Add a few strawberries, if in season.
You can swap this for any 4-GiP cereal of your choice (see tables, page 283).
OR
2 thin slices toasted raisin bread, topped with sautéed mushrooms, optional: sliced mushrooms sautéed in 10 sprays of oil and sprinkled with dried herbs. Throw in some fresh garlic if you like.

Mid-morning booster

Tomato and mustard bruschetta: 1 Warburtons All In One Roll
topped with Tomato and Mustard Seed Salad (mix together
10 halved cherry tomatoes, 1 tsp coarse-grained mustard, a
handful of chopped parsley and 1–2 tbsp balsamic vinegar).
OR
10 shells of roasted peanuts.

Lunch

**Sunday Roast: 3 slices of lean roast beef, or 3 slices roast
chicken breast, or 1 roast chicken leg, thigh or drumstick
(skinless), or 3 slices roast pork, or 2 slices roast turkey,
or 2 slices lean roast lamb.**

**1 small sweet potato, or 4 new potatoes in their skins,
boiled and then sprayed with oil and roasted separately
in the oven.**

**Unlimited fat-free cabbage, spinach, broccoli, celeriac,
courgettes, fennel, leeks, marrow, peppers, turnip,
spring greens or any other GiP-free vegetables (see
tables, page 293).**

1–2 tbsp instant gravy (do not use juices from the meat).
OR
Spinach and Ricotta Cannelloni (see recipe, page 264).
GiP-free roasted vegetables: mix together your favourite
combination of chopped peppers, mushrooms, onions,
courgettes, asparagus, celery, baby corn and tomatoes.
Add a teaspoon or so of crushed garlic, a sprig of
rosemary or dried herbs, a little salt and pepper. Place in a

foil-lined tray and bake in a hot oven till cooked, about 15–20 minutes.

Spiced Pear with Ginger Fromage Frais: soften a quartered pear in 5 sprays of oil and a little lemon juice over a medium heat. Flavour with ground cinnamon. Mix a pinch of ginger powder with 50 ml virtually fat-free fromage frais and serve this with the warm pears, decorated with fresh mint and a dusting of icing sugar.

Quick fix: The oven is on for the cannelloni anyway, so today's meal includes a speedy roasted vegetable recipe as an accompaniment. If you like, make some extra so that you can have a roasted vegetable sandwich for lunch tomorrow.

Mid-afternoon pick-me-up

2 satsumas.

OR

1 rich tea biscuit with hot drink using milk from allowance.

Dinner

Have a quick 'n' light supper today:

Chilli beans on toast: ½ can of chilli beans on a slice of seeded or multigrain toast.

Unlimited GiP-free salad vegetables with 1 tbsp of fat-free dressing.

1 diet yoghurt (as it is or enjoy it frozen into a sorbet-type dessert. Defrost about 30 minutes or so before eating or freeze for about 4 hours if you prefer a frozen yoghurt texture).

OR

Unsweetened apple juice, 150 ml.

Prawn cocktail: 125 g cooked prawns dressed in 1–2 tbsp fat-free Thousand Island dressing, served on a bed of mixed salad leaves and diced cucumber.

Serve with 1 slice of Burgen soya and linseed bread spread lightly with a coarse-grain mustard.

3 plums.

Evening comforter (optional)

1 oatcake with a hot drink using milk from allowance.

OR

8–10 grapes.

Step 3: Get GiP Fit (day 6)

Remember, you may combine these into one 20-minute burst if you prefer.

a) Fitness Burst 1: 10 mins in the morning or at lunchtime

Stand to attention! Today's first 10-minute burst is marching on the spot.

b) Fitness Burst 2: 10 mins at lunchtime or in the evening

Try a gentle jog for Fitness Burst 2. If you're able, go outside so that you get some fresh air. You could do it at lunchtime or later in the day.

My GI Tip: Following an exercise session, refuel with low-GI carbohydrates. This allows your body to continue to burn fat but replaces those essential carbohydrate stores in the body needed for exercise.

Dr Emma Stevenson, University of Nottingham

Weight-bearing exercise (and that includes walking up stairs or a gentle slope) improves bone density, therefore delaying the onset of osteoporosis, especially in later life. It's never too late to start. Seek professional guidance first.

Step 4: Time in, time out (day 6)

Your two-minute springboard!

Go to the *Practical Tools* section (page 354) and list your three achievements for today.

Tiffin Box

Choose tomorrow's menu items so you can be prepared:

Tomorrow's lunch offers you a chance to be smart with your leftovers from today. Any roast meat or roasted vegetables can be speedily conjured up into a sandwich or a tortilla wrap for tomorrow. If there are no leftovers, you might decide to opt for some sushi from the local sandwich bar. You might want to prepare an Olive and Cucumber Snack Box, page 226, either for lunch or for one of your snacks. This and the GiP-free Veg Box (page 226) are very handy for hunger quick-fixes. If you are going out to work get the dried fruits and drinks ready to slip into your bag as you swing out of the door tomorrow.

Take a 'Me Moment'

We tend to feel full a little while after we have eaten enough, just as we tend to feel thirsty after we've become dehydrated. At intervals throughout the day, rate your hunger on the scale under *Practical Tools* (page 355) to start getting in tune with your appetite and satiety (fullness) cues.

As today draws to a close, allow yourself a few minutes to feel a magnificent sense of peace and calm engulf you. You can do this by allowing your imagination to go to a special place where you have experienced these feelings before and recreate them in your mind's eye.

Power Tips

❑ Every healthy thought you have leads to a healthy food choice. Thoughts are like drips of water falling on stone. Over time they carve deep channels.

❑ Chew your food slowly, putting your cutlery down between mouthfuls. Serve yourself a smaller amount of food and take 15 minutes to eat it. You might find that when you eat slowly, you will be satisfied much earlier.

❑ The Department of Health recommends five 30-minute
sessions of moderate-intensity activity each week.
Getting GiP-fit helps you to reach these levels without it
being a slog!

❑ People sometimes accomplish the impossible. They weren't
necessarily the most outstanding humans. They just had a
hugely compelling desire to succeed. You can too!

DAY 7 (MONDAY)

Step 1: Today's Energiser

Snakes and ladders!

Have fun playing our uniquely adapted board game. What do your answers reveal? This is a gentle reminder that each choice you make has its own set of consequences. This is not to say what's right or wrong, simply that if you want to get to the top of the board successfully by day 10, there are certain choices you will be motivated to make to ensure this specific outcome is met.

Q1 *Do you eat breakfast?*

❑ **Yes.** Great choice. You are consciously nourishing your body and therefore your mind, to manage the day ahead resourcefully. This in turn will keep your energy and motivational levels high. **Move up several rungs on the ladder.**

❑ **No.** You are not taking care of yourself. Follow this plan and notice your energy and motivational levels rise. This in turn will keep you upbeat and more likely to succeed with any goal. One step at a time leads to a positive accumulative effect for the best! **Move down a small snake.**

❑ **Sometimes.** This 10-day diet helps you to understand how eating a low-GI breakfast will nourish your body and mind. Do what you need to do to ensure you eat the recommended meals. You know you're worth it! **Move up a couple of rungs on the ladder.**

Q2 *How often do you give yourself permission to take a 'Me Moment'?*

- ❏ **Daily.** Good on you. You clearly appreciate that looking after yourself means that you can take care of others effectively while keeping yourself uplifted. **Move up several rungs on the ladder.**
- ❏ **Never.** Less is more! By allowing yourself the time and space to slow down, you are likelier to be much more productive in other areas of your life. Give it a go. **Move down a small snake.**
- ❏ **Occasionally.** You'll already know and feel the benefits of giving yourself permission to experience this precious time. Commit to finding a few minutes in your life, daily. You know it makes sense! **Move up a few rungs on the ladder or one small ladder.**

Q3 *How often do you drink alcohol?*

- ❏ **Occasionally.** Your body is a temple and sometimes it's a nightclub! If you're watching your weight, it's best to have no more than seven units of alcohol a week and to make sure you have a few alcohol-free days as well. Research shows that a glass of red wine with meals may protect your heart. **Move up a couple of rungs on the ladder.**
- ❏ **Never.** How great to wake up every day with a clear head and no regrets from the night before! No extra cals

to fret over either. Bonus! **Move up a couple of rungs on the ladder.**

❑ **Often.** Your body seems to have turned into a permanent nightclub! You're out of balance. Distraction works well. Make a list of what is effective and try it (you can use the *Practical Tools* section, page 359, for this list). Before you indulge in that extra drink, ask yourself what need you're trying to fulfil and deal with it in a healthy and resourceful way.
Move down a snake.

Q4 *How regularly do you take physical activity?*

❑ **Daily – at least two bursts of 10 minutes.**
Great! Regular exercise has so many benefits. In addition to keeping the body and mind healthy, burning off the cals and toning the muscles, it includes uplifting the spirits, keeping motivational levels up and warding off depression.
Move up several rungs on the ladder.

❑ **Sometimes, when I feel like it.** Exercise is one of the most effective ways of nourishing your mind and body (which are inextricably linked). Just two 10-minute bursts of moderate-intensity physical activity daily can have significant benefits. Build it in to your lifestyle. **Move up a few rungs on the ladder.**

❑ **Couch potatoes don't!** Use it or lose it! It is well known you can't shift the cals from the comfort of your armchair, so get going on a regular routine that you can enjoy and that you can effortlessly fit into your lifestyle. You'll start to notice the difference quickly. **Move down a snake.**

Q5 *I consciously choose low-GI carbs...*

☐ **At every meal.** Celebrate your choices. What you choose today will bring long-term rewards in terms of health, fitness and inch loss. **Move up several rungs on the ladder.**

☐ **Sometimes.** Remember that the choices you make have an accumulative effect. By making low-GI carbs your daily choice, you'll appreciate an overall sense of lasting energy and a feel-good state, which will also increase your sense of motivation. **Move up a few rungs on the ladder.**

☐ **Too much like hard work!** Choose differently! Give yourself an extra boost of motivation. Focus on the end result and how you will look and feel. Direct your thoughts in that direction only. Failure is not an option! Try the VVPC plate method which will help you to choose low-GI foods automatically (see GiP Rule 4 in Chapter 1, *GI and the Gi Plan*). **Move down a snake.**

Q6 *Do you snack out?*

☐ **Yes. But only the low-GI ones as recommended.** Pat yourself on the back. Low-GI snacks and meals help to sustain your energy levels throughout the day. **Move up several rungs on the ladder.**

☐ **Some days, when I get home starving, I make straight for anything snackie in the fridge.** Often this happens when you've not had enough to eat at lunch or have missed a mid-afternoon snack. Be prepared by having a GiP-free Veg Box (see recipe, page 226) in the fridge, or sit down to have a planned snack after work. **Move down a snake.**

❏ **Yes, the naughty but nice ones like crisps and chocolates.** Your future starts here. If your current sense of wellness and feelings about yourself are not what you would wish them to be, doing and eating as you've always done can only bring you more of the same. Make up your mind to make these small changes here and now. The results will be worth it! **Move down a snake.**

Q7 *Imagine it is now day 12. Having achieved your 10-day goal, how will you go about sustaining it?*

❏ **My low-GI plan is now part of my new lifestyle. Sustaining it is effortless.** Congratulations! You've achieved what you set out to achieve. Whenever you need to, remind yourself of the rewards this new healthy lifestyle brings. **Move up to the very top of the board.**

❏ **I am confident that I'll keep to the general principles although I may fall down occasionally.** If you do, simply pick up on the low-GI choices the next day. You already know your new lifestyle is worth it. **Move up close to the top of the board.**

❏ **I was only in it for the quick fix! Now I've seen the benefits, I'll keep it up.** Acting out of these tried and tested well-informed choices today will shape your future. Celebrate your commitment to carry on. Take a look at your achievements under *Practical Tools* (page 354). **Move up several rungs of the ladder, near to the top.**

Step 2: Select Your Menu (day 7)

Your meal plan is based on a daily target of 17 GiPs, split
on average as follows:

Breakfast:	4 GiPs
Mid-morning booster:	2 GiPs
Lunch:	5 GiPs
Mid-afternoon pick-me-up:	1 GiP
Dinner:	4 GiPs
Evening comforter:	1 GiP

You don't need to count the GiPs; it's all been done for you.

You can make your own menus using the GiP tables so long as
you keep to these amounts.

You can have unlimited amounts of GiP-free veg (see table,
page 293), including as much as you like of the GiP-free
recipes (page 199).

For drinks throughout the day: 200 ml (⅓ pint) skimmed or
semi-skimmed milk, unlimited herbal teas, unsweetened tea
and coffee, sugar-free drinks, water.

For lunch: These suggestions are low GI, filling and varied. You will
be preparing most the previous evening. If some days you can't
be bothered, you can opt for a low- or medium-GI sandwich
from Marks & Spencer's 'Count on Us' range (check labels), a
Sainsbury's GI-tested sandwich (see tables, page 281) or a tailor-
made sandwich from a sandwich bar using our suggested low-GI
ingredients (see *Getting Ready for Day One*, page 43). You are
more likely to get results with the suggested lunches here.

The evening comforter is optional. If you don't like evening snacks, have the comforter at any other time of the day.

Men – have an extra 3 GiPs each day. Check out the tables at the back for GiP values of everyday foods.

Breakfast

4 tbsp muesli with 200 ml (⅓ pint) skimmed or semi-skimmed milk.
You can swap this for any 4-GiP cereal of your choice (see tables, page 283).

> *My GI Tip: Keeping to a low-GI diet has worked wonders for my health. I eat porridge, wholegrain toast or wholegrain cereal most mornings and this sets me up for the day. I've lost weight with my new healthy lifestyle change, which in turn has given me even better energy levels.*
> ANTONY WORRALL THOMPSON, CELEBRITY CHEF

OR

1 scrambled egg: made with a little milk, seasoning, and scrambled in about ½ tsp of olive oil.
1 slice multigrain bread, toasted.
Grilled tomato halves, optional.
1 Tesco Probiotic Original Drink (low GI).

No time for breakfast before you leave the house for work? Have it at work… Try a 4-GiP cereal.

Mid-morning booster

15 g treat-size white or milk chocolate bar or a piece of fruit.
Sugar-free cold drink, or hot drink using milk from allowance.
OR
Mug of lentil soup (bought or home-made) or up to 20 olives.

Lunch

Small single portion sushi (6 mini-sushi).
Olive and Cucumber Snack box (throw together 10 black or
green olives, cucumber sticks, and any combination of the
following: celery sticks, radishes, pickled onions, gherkins,
water chestnuts).
1 pot of reduced-fat mousse.
1 fresh apple.

*Did you know that masters of sushi-making will attempt
to get the rice grains facing in the same direction?*

OR
Use up your leftovers:
Meat sandwich made from Sunday's leftover roast meat:
2 slices of Burgen soya and linseed bread, spread with
yeast extract (e.g. Marmite) or mustard, filled with piles of
rocket salad, sliced peppers, and 2–3 slices of lean roast
meat seasoned with pepper and any herbs of your choice.
1 firm pear.
Veg sandwich made from Sunday's leftover roasted vegetables:
two slices of Warburtons All In One, or granary bread or a
tortilla wrap, spread with yeast extract (e.g. Marmite) or
mustard, filled with masses of roasted vegetables and

seasoned with pepper and any herbs of your choice. (You
can use any bread up to the value of 3.5 GiPs.)
1 satsuma.

Fat squeezer: Yeast extract makes a B-vitamin rich
and fat-free spread for sandwiches. But don't add any
salt, there's plenty there already.

Mid-afternoon pick-me-up

1 oatcake or 1 triangle Jacob Essentials – Wholewheat
   cracker with sesame seeds & rosemary.
Hot drink using milk from allowance.
OR
Reduced-fat chocolate milk shake made from 200 ml (⅓ pint)
   skimmed milk and 2 tsp Nesquik milk shake powder.

Dinner

Chargrilled salmon steak: flavour a medium-sized salmon steak
   with your favourite herbs, a drizzle of balsamic vinegar, a
   touch of fresh garlic, and grill under a medium heat.
3 small new potatoes in their skins, boiled (add some mint for
   flavour).
Unlimited roasted GiP-free
   vegetables (see table,
   page 293, for examples,
   or GiP-free recipes,
   page 199).
12 strawberries.

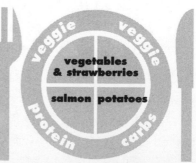

OR

GiP-free Tomato Soup with Crunchy Onions and Green
  Pepper 'Croutons' (see recipe, page 200).

Baked Flat Mushrooms with Melted Camembert (see recipe,
  page 252).

Unlimited roasted GiP-free vegetables (see table, page 293,
  for examples, or GiP-free recipes, page 199), optional.

I fresh satsuma.

Tonight's dinner uses an 'eat-now-eat-later' concept.
Save some GiP-free vegetable leftovers for your ricotta
cheese and roasted veg rolls tomorrow.

Evening comforter (optional)

I diet yoghurt.

OR

I triangle Jacob Essentials – Wholewheat cracker with
  sesame seeds & rosemary.

Hot drink using milk from allowance.

Step 3: Get GiP Fit (day 7)

Remember, you may combine these into one 20-minute burst
if you prefer.

a) Fitness Burst I: 10 mins in the morning or at lunchtime
Your choice. There are several ideas to pick from. If you've
tended to do mainly brisk walking perhaps today is the time to

try something different? Ideas include marching on the spot, swimming, dancing, stair work, cycling or jogging.

b) Fitness Burst 2: 10 mins at lunchtime or in the evening
Once again, it's your preference but perhaps choose differently to Burst 1 if you haven't gone for the 20-minute option.

Remember, stretch means tension not pain.

Step 4: Time in, time out (day 7)

Your two-minute springboard!

Go to the *Practical Tools* section (page 354) and list your three achievements for today.

Tiffin Box

Choose tomorrow's menu items so you can be prepared:

If you're going for boiled eggs in the morning, you might want to save yourself some time by boiling the eggs tonight. Then you need simply crack or peel the cooked eggs and reheat in the microwave tomorrow.

If you prepared roasted vegetables tonight, then any leftovers can be used for tomorrow's ricotta cheese and roasted vegetable rolls. Alternatively, the tuna and cucumber pitta pocket can be prepared in a matter of minutes. The baby sweetcorn and chive salad is created by simply throwing a few ingredients together and makes a tasty GiP-free accompaniment.

Now's a good time to get your Olive and Cucumber Snack Box (page 226) ready and to make sure you have the fruits and nuts to hand for the morning.

Take a 'Me Moment'

Spread a little happiness: Your body has its own natural and sophisticated pharmacy of 'happy' chemicals, such as endorphins, that it calls on as and when required. Try this.

- ☐ Remember a time when you felt totally happy, contented, calm and at peace with yourself.

- ☐ What do you see, hear and feel?

- ☐ See the picture clearly and in colour. Make it brighter, pump up the volume of sounds and increase the intensity of the feelings.

- ☐ Consider where in your body this feeling of happiness lies. If it were to have a colour, what colour would it be?

- ☐ Now, move the colour up and down your entire body from the tips of your toes to the top of your head, making it brighter each time.

- ☐ Feel the glow and inner radiation caused by the release of these natural 'happy' chemicals as they spread throughout your body.

- ☐ Repeat this exercise several times by recalling the same or other happy experiences to naturally boost these chemicals.

Power Tips

☐ Give yourself an hour and notice the high energy levels you feel after your low-GI meal. Use this extra energy to accomplish something on today's 'to do' list.

☐ Beans are a low-GI wonder food. Experiment by throwing them into salads, soups, casseroles and curries. All you need to do is open a can or put them in a slow cooker.

☐ Remaining physically active outdoors, in different types of weather and terrain, makes for a more challenging and enjoyable workout.

☐ Rather than thinking about losing 10 pounds, think about shedding one pound, ten times!

DAY 8 (TUESDAY)

Step 1: Today's Energiser

Overcoming stress – take the test

Here is a simple quiz to help you find out what is draining your energy. The quiz features a list of some of the areas in your life that may be causing you stress. Have a go to get more insight into the factors causing you unnecessary stress pangs. You can use the results to help you to make necessary changes in your life. Take a few deep breaths, clear your mind and off you go. Tick off the items that are applicable to you.

Each item you tick is worth 4 per cent. The highest level of stress you can score is 100 per cent. Add up your percentage points.

Give consideration to where you can make immediate changes, no matter how small.

Every so often, take the test again to see if your stress level has lowered. For instance, let's say that when you first did the test, you scored 80 per cent and then two months later you made some changes in your life to help reduce your stress level and you scored 70 per cent. This means that you lowered your stress level by 10 per cent, and that means that some of the changes you have made in your life are working.

My Environment

____ I do not live in a secure environment.

_____ I would like to change my home environment.

_____ My home is untidy.

_____ I have a lot of distractions (such as watching too much TV).

_____ My home needs some TLC.

My Mind, Body and Spirit

_____ I eat unhealthy food.

_____ I have low self-esteem.

_____ I lack spiritual development and nourishment.

_____ I feel demotivated.

_____ I do not nurture my health.

My Relationships

_____ I need to forgive.

_____ I am holding on to grudges.

_____ I am angry with someone.

_____ I am in a dysfunctional relationship.

_____ I need to resolve an issue with someone close.

My Finances

_____ I spend more than I make.

_____ I am in debt.

_____ I don't have a future plan for my finances.

_____ I can barely pay my bills.

_____ I have a bad credit rating.

My Career/Business

_____ I do not enjoy my work.

___ I do not feel fulfilled in my present career.

___ I am in a dead-end job.

___ I have a business idea but don't follow it through.

___ I let fear stand in the way of my moving up the career ladder.

If you have joined the human race, chances are that there are times when you feel stressed, busy, unfulfilled, bored, rushed, under the weather, overworked, underpaid, irritable and frustrated – hopefully not all at the same time! However, consider this. There is no such thing as stress, only stressful thoughts. The meaning that you give to something ultimately determines your experience. In other words, what you focus your thoughts on is what causes you to feel the way you do. So ban those negative thoughts from your mind!

Stress is a major contributor to comfort eating, drinking and bingeing, and is responsible for many illnesses. Being ill-at-ease with yourself could be thought of as being 'dis-eased'. Make up your mind today to be happy with who you are. This way you are less likely to punish yourself by overindulging.

❑ Decide how you would recognise balance in your life.

❑ Consider what you would see, hear and feel.

❑ Choose some specific and tangible actions that will support you in achieving this.

❑ Notice what's working or not, as the case may be, and make appropriate changes.

❑ Celebrate all your success along the way, no matter how small. It's the cumulative result that counts!

Step 2: Select Your Menu (day 8)

Your meal plan is based on a daily target of 17 GiPs, split on average as follows:

Breakfast:	4 GiPs
Mid-morning booster:	2 GiPs
Lunch:	5 GiPs
Mid-afternoon pick-me-up:	1 GiP
Dinner:	4 GiPs
Evening comforter:	1 GiP

You don't need to count the GiPs; it's all been done for you.

You can make your own menus using the GiP tables so long as you keep to these amounts.

You can have unlimited amounts of GiP-free veg (see table, page 293), including as much as you like of the GiP-free recipes (page 199).

For drinks throughout the day: 200 ml (⅓ pint) skimmed or semi-skimmed milk, unlimited herbal teas, unsweetened tea and coffee, sugar-free drinks, water.

For lunch: These suggestions are low GI, filling and varied. You will be preparing most the previous evening. If some days you can't be bothered, you can opt for a low- or medium-GI sandwich from Marks & Spencer's 'Count on Us' range (check labels), a Sainsbury's GI-tested sandwich (see tables, page 281) or a tailor-made sandwich from a sandwich bar using our suggested low-GI ingredients (see *Getting Ready for Day One*, page 43). You are more likely to get results with the suggested lunches here.

The evening comforter is optional. If you don't like evening snacks, have the comforter at any other time of the day.

Men – have an extra 3 GiPs each day. Check out the tables at the back for GiP values of everyday foods.

Breakfast

Glass of unsweetened fruit juice (150 ml).
1 slice multigrain bread, toasted, with a scraping of half-fat
    unsaturated or low-fat spread.
1 tsp reduced-sugar jam.
You can swap this for any 4-GiP cereal of your choice (see tables, page 283).

OR

2 boiled eggs or try fried eggs cooked in 10 sprays of oil, covered and cooked in the hot steam over a low heat.
Fresh or canned tomatoes, if desired.
1 slice granary toast.
Scraping of half-fat unsaturated or low-fat spread or yeast extract.

No time for breakfast? Have a 180 ml carton of (low-Gi) innocent kids Oranges, Mangoes and Pineapples with 2 oatcakes on the train or at work.

Mid-morning booster

5 tbsp All Bran with 200 ml (⅓ pt) skimmed or semi-skimmed milk
OR
Handful of peanuts in shells (10 shells).

> *My GI Tip: I always carry a bag of nuts and some fruit around with me and don't let myself get to that low-blood-sugar stage where I crave Krispy Kremes! (Doesn't always work though.)*
>
> CHARLOTTE HAIGH, HEALTH JOURNALIST

Lunch

Ricotta cheese and roasted vegetable rolls: 2 Warburtons
  All In One Rolls, filled with 100 g ricotta cheese and
  masses of GiP-free Roasted Veg (from previous day's
  leftovers or from recipe, page 217) and fresh basil leaves.
  Use simple salad vegetables if you prefer. Add some
  chopped red peppers.
1 fresh apple or 10 olives.

Ricotta cheese here gives you moisture and flavour
without piling on the calories.

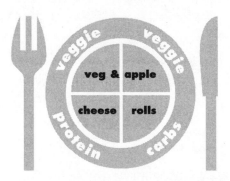

OR

Tuna and cucumber pitta pocket: half a pitta bread, filled with
  tuna and cucumber mix (½ can drained tuna in brine,

diced cucumber, freshly chopped dill, dressed in fat-free
Thousand Island dressing).

Handful of cherry tomatoes.

GiP-free baby sweetcorn and chive salad (mix together a can
of drained baby sweetcorn, a handful of snipped chives
and a drizzle of lemon juice. Season with salt and pepper.)

1 fun-size Snickers bar or 15 g milk chocolate bar.

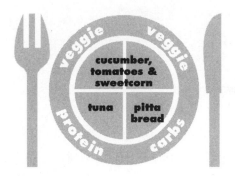

Mid-afternoon pick-me-up

Vie Shot Apple/Carrot/Strawberry.

OR

Olive and Cucumber Snack Box (throw together 10 black or
green olives, cucumber sticks, and any combination of
the following: celery sticks, radishes, pickled onions,
gherkins, water chestnuts).

1 satsuma.

Dinner

Take away/ready meal low-GI quick-fix choices are fine once a
week. Try these…

Pizza night: 2 slices from a medium (22 cm/9 in diameter)

deep-pan or thin-based pizza. Ask for less cheese and
more vegetables. Masses of crispy lettuce, tomatoes,
cucumber, celery, spring onion, dressed in fat-free dressing.
1 Tesco Healthy Living Light Peach and Apricot yoghurt (low GI)

OR

Ready meal: 1 portion of Sainsbury's Be Good to Yourself
Chicken Tikka Masala and Rice.
6 sliced peaches canned in juice.

Evening comforter (optional)

5 ready-to-eat prunes.

OR

Diet hot chocolate made up from a sachet with water or
skimmed milk.

Step 3: Get GiP Fit (day 8)

Remember, you may combine these into one 20-minute burst
if you prefer.

a) Fitness Burst 1: 10 mins in the morning or at lunchtime
Go for the stairs in your Fitness Burst 1. Ten minutes of
walking up and down stairs will do it. Alternatively, use the
bottom step as an 'aerobic stepper'. Simply step up – first with
your right foot and then your left – and then step down –
right foot first, then left – and repeat, for 10 minutes or as long
as you can manage. It's aerobic (and therefore fat-burning) and
also 'weight bearing', so it strengthens the bones. It's easy and

you can listen to music at the same time so it doesn't get boring. Throughout the day, continue to make a conscious effort to use the stairs.

b) Fitness Burst 2: 10 mins at lunchtime or in the evening
Plan to go for a jog in your lunch break or later in the day.

Always seek opportunities to choose an active option.

Step 4: Time in, time out (day 8)

Your two-minute springboard!

Go to the *Practical Tools* section (page 354) and list your three achievements for today.

Tiffin Box

Choose tomorrow's menu items so you can be prepared:

Your GiP-free Veg Box may by now have become a regular habit. Think about varying the contents of your box so you have a bit more variety for tomorrow. Check out the GiP-free vegetables in the tables at the back of this book (page 293).

Decide on whether you are tempted by the filling Potato, Apple and Tuna Salad (page 243) or would prefer to have a roast beef sandwich. The salad will take about as much time as it takes to boil or microwave 4 new potatoes – you can be draining the tuna and chopping the apple while the potatoes are cooking. The sandwich can either be prepared at home this evening, or you could buy one tomorrow. Flick back to the guidance on bought sandwiches (page 61) so you can go for a lower-GI option. Get your convenient snack item ready so you are on track tomorrow.

Take a 'Me Moment'

Wise men have said over time that when you smile you release a sweet substance that nourishes your whole body. Conversely, when you feel negative you release harmful chemicals that clog up your flow of energy.

Bring the classic pose of the Buddha to mind. See his smile. It seems to radiate both inwardly and out.

Model this. Smile from the inside out. Allow the smile into your eyes so that they twinkle and sparkle. Let it stretch to your ears.

Allow the sense of good feeling to travel around the rest of your body.

Relax even more and bathe in the essence of the feel-good factor as it spreads everywhere.

Enjoy the stillness and serenity this brings. Remain in this pose for a few minutes.

Life is right!

Power Tips

❑ Make time to do the things you enjoy and find more of the simple pleasures in life.

❑ Fed up with drinking water and missing the fizzy stuff? Simply add some sparkling water to your favourite sugar-free cordial, throw in a sprig of mint, some ice and some fresh lime wedges and you have a GiP-free fruity fizzy drink.

❑ Build in activity that fits easily into your everyday way of life, so that it becomes an effortless routine and one that you look forward to. Aim to increase the time, over time.

❑ You are part of a world that views being busy as a status symbol – diary envy! Choose to just 'be' and enjoy the chill-out space that is needed to nourish you.

DAY 9 (WEDNESDAY)

Step 1: Today's Energiser

Friends, who needs 'em?

Have you ever noticed how those closest to you influence different parts of your personality? This happens because you are influenced by the company you keep. The same is true for the goals you set. Do you know of a little angel who goes off to school and, after a while, returns with enough swear words to make a trooper cringe? Mix with critical people and you learn to be one of them. Mix with an enthusiastic crowd and that rubs off on you too. Spend time with those who value their health and wellbeing and you'll find yourself doing the same. By choosing to be with friends and/or family who want to support, nourish and nurture you, you'll boost your will to succeed even more.

Action point

Surround yourself with good company and tell 'em how much you appreciate them!

Step 2: Select Your Menu (day 9)

Your meal plan is based on a daily target of 17 GiPs, split on average as follows:

Breakfast:	4 GiPs
Mid-morning booster:	2 GiPs

Lunch:	5 GiPs
Mid-afternoon pick-me-up:	1 GiP
Dinner:	4 GiPs
Evening comforter:	1 GiP

You don't need to count the GiPs; it's all been done for you.

You can make your own menus using the GiP tables so long as you keep to these amounts.

You can have unlimited amounts of GiP-free veg (see table, page 293), including as much as you like of the GiP-free recipes (page 199).

For drinks throughout the day: 200 ml (⅓ pint) skimmed or semi-skimmed milk, unlimited herbal teas, unsweetened tea and coffee, sugar-free drinks, water.

For lunch: These suggestions are low GI, filling and varied. You will be preparing most the previous evening. If some days you can't be bothered, you can opt for a low- or medium-GI sandwich from Marks & Spencer's 'Count on Us' range (check labels), a Sainsbury's GI-tested sandwich (see tables, page 281) or a tailor-made sandwich from a sandwich bar using our suggested low-GI ingredients (see *Getting Ready for Day One*, page 43). You are more likely to get results with the suggested lunches here.

The evening comforter is optional. If you don't like evening snacks, have the comforter at any other time of the day.

Men – have an extra 3 GiPs each day. Check out the tables at the back for GiP values of everyday foods.

Breakfast

2 tsp peanut butter on 1 slice of bread or toast.
OR
4 tbsp muesli with 200 ml (⅓ pint) skimmed or semi-
skimmed milk.
*You can swap this for any 4-GiP cereal of your choice (see tables,
page 283).*

Mid-morning booster

GiP-free Veg Box (throw together any combination of the
following: courgette sticks, cucumber sticks, baby
gherkins, radishes, cherry tomatoes, celery, baby
sweetcorn, sugar snap peas, pickled onions, peppers).
2 tbsp half-fat hummus
OR
1 rich tea biscuit with a hot drink using milk from allowance.

Lunch

Potato, Apple and Tuna salad (see recipe, page 243).
Substitute the tuna for a large boiled egg if you prefer a
vegetarian option.
12 cherries or 6 sliced peaches canned in juice.

*Massive salad for hungry days. Cold potatoes have a
lower GI than freshly cooked ones.*

OR
Roast beef and mustard sandwich: 2 slices multigrain bread,
moistened with a spread of mustard instead of butter,

2 slices lean roast beef and plenty of salad vegetables. Either make this at home or ask for a personalised low-GiP sandwich at a sandwich bar.

Glass of tomato juice, flavoured with mint or Worcester sauce, if desired.

Mid-afternoon pick-me-up

Mug of minestrone soup, made from a sachet.

1 oatcake or 1 triangle Jacob Essentials – Wholewheat cracker with sesame seeds & rosemary.

OR

1 diet yoghurt.

Dinner

Lemony Cod Strips with Spicy Bulgur Wheat (see recipe, page 248).

Unlimited steamed broccoli.

Chargrilled beef tomatoes: cut 2 tomatoes in half, drizzle with soy sauce and grill till charred.

8–10 grapes or Instant (Fresh) Cherry Cheesecake (see recipe, page 273).

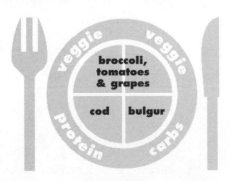

Steaming doesn't mean using special machines or gadgets. Simply put around 1 cm (½ in) water into a pan with the vegetables. Cover with a tight-fitting lid, cook quickly until just cooked but not too soft over a high heat, and drain. If you leave cooked vegetables lying around, they will lose some of their nutrients, so serve immediately.

OR

Garlic Spaghetti with Courgette Ribbons (see recipe, page 258).

Sautéed chestnut mushrooms: spray a generous handful of chestnut mushrooms with 5 sprays of oil, some dried herbs and seasoning, and microwave or stir-fry.

GiP-free tossed green salad: mix together your favourite green salad vegetables such as crispy lettuce, rocket, baby spinach, watercress, celery and cucumber. Throw in some chopped herbs such as flat-leaf parsley or coriander and flavour with lime or lemon juice. Season to taste.

I fresh apricot.

Feel like having an ice lolly? Then freeze some sugar-free squash in an ice lolly maker and enjoy at your leisure.

Evening comforter (optional)

Mug of Marmite or other yeast extract.

I rich tea biscuit.

OR

Dip 'n' sticks: 2 tbsp Tzatziki with celery and pepper sticks.

Step 3: Get GiP Fit (day 9)

Remember, you may combine these into one 20-minute burst if you prefer.

a) Fitness Burst 1: 10 mins in the morning or at lunchtime
Start today with a jog. Remember you can do this for 20 minutes if you wish to complete the required physical activity in one burst.

b) Fitness Burst 2: 10 mins at lunchtime or in the evening
Treat yourself to a swim. It may be possible for you to fit in a short 10 minutes during your lunch break or later in the day. Alternatively, you could allow yourself a full 20 minutes to complete today's fitness requirement.

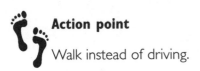

Action point
Walk instead of driving.

Step 4: Time in, time out (day 9)

Your two-minute springboard!

Go to the *Practical Tools* section (page 354) and list your three achievements for today.

Tiffin Box

Choose tomorrow's menu items so you can be prepared. Tomorrow may be the last day of your lower-GI eating plan, or it may just be the end of your first stepping stone towards a longer-term healthier lifestyle. Whatever your desires, be certain that if you've kept to the eating plans as suggested in this book, you are already living the lower-GI lifestyle, with all the benefits it has to offer. By now, you will probably have got into the habit of adding vegetables and salads to your meals, of eating dried fruit or a handful of nuts between meals, and of choosing lower-fat, lower-GI cooking methods.

Have a glance at tomorrow's lunch and remember that you are now equipped to swap the suggested choices with any other 5-GiP lunch of your choice. Either select a menu, create your own lunch using the tables at the back, or simply flick through the previous day's lunch choices and choose something that tempts your taste buds today. Spend your 10 minutes of preparation time so that you're sure to be in charge of what's on your plate tomorrow.

If you're able to make toast in the daytime, you could go for the omega-3 rich sardines on toast (or use canned mackerel or pilchards). Or try the egg and tomato roll – you may already have some of these rolls in your freezer if you took on the handy hints in a previous chapter.

Get the Olive and Cucumber Snack Box, fruit, yoghurt and/or nuts ready so you don't need to prepare them in the morning. Do you have all the ingredients for tomorrow's tapas selection or pan-fried turkey?

Enjoy it, you are nearly there…

Take a 'Me Moment'

Ask yourself who would make a great role model? And, commit to spending time with them.

What characteristics have they got? List them on paper or mentally.

You can only recognise in others what you already have, at some level, in yourself.

What can you do to develop these more?

Commit to doing so here and now!

Here's an example of a mother, wishing to increase her sense of fun and playfulness, who chose to model the child-like qualities of her 12-year-old daughter:

'No matter what's on her mind, my 12-year-old is forever bouncing around the place. She just can't sit still. There is an inherent energy whenever you observe her and she appears to smile with her whole body. During conversation, she is attentive, smiling and all there for me. Yet, there's always a slight bounce to her movements and that adds a beautiful child-like response to any question I may ask.

'Although this bouncy exterior isn't all that makes her as wonderful as she is, I find that when I take on that bounciness or spring in my own step, I too can be a little bit more relaxed about all the trials and tribulations around me. I learn to take life a little less seriously. Simple things like rolling around on the floor with her help me to enjoy our moments together and help me to be more in touch with that fun side of me that often gets locked away while I wear the mother, housewife and career-woman hat. I try to carry her image with me and remember her lightness and charm as often as I can.'

Power Tips

❏ Make a conscious effort to spend more time with people who laugh a lot, play a lot and who value their wellness. It will soon rub off!

❏ Generally, the more natural a food is, the lower will be its GI value. Compare wholegrain flour to refined white flour, porridge to cornflakes, or brown rice to instant rice. Start looking at a food and thinking about it before you eat it.

❏ Try ice-skating or roller-blading. You'll laugh a lot, boosting your happy chemicals, while toning your bottom, thighs and stomach.

❏ It's official! Even one really good friend can boost your immune system.

DAY 10 (THURSDAY)

Step 1: Today's Energiser

Wheel of Fortune

Of course, you make your own good fortune. This is largely down to how you think about things and the meaning you give to any set of events and circumstances. You will already know of people who are never satisfied, no matter how much they have or acquire in various aspects of their life. And yet, there are others who seem to have very little, who delight in the simplicity of what they do have and those they have to share it with. When you are able to find a positive perspective on anything, you will have the mindset that enables you to seek some degree of growth or learning, no matter how adverse a situation might appear on the surface.

Take the farmer in the following example:

A father and his son owned a farm. One day the only horse they had ran away.
'What terrible, bad luck,' the neighbours cried.
'Good luck, bad luck, who knows?' said the farmer.

Several weeks later the horse returned, bringing with him three wild mares.
'What excellent luck,' said the neighbours.
'Good luck, bad luck, who knows?' replied the farmer.

The son began to ride the wild horses and one day he was thrown off and broke his leg.
'What bad luck,' said the neighbours.

'Good luck, bad luck,' replied the farmer in his enigmatic manner, 'who knows?'

The following week the army came to the village to take all the young men to war. The farmer's son was still disabled with his injury and so was spared.

Good luck, bad luck, who knows?

The Wheel of Fortune is a refection of your personal vision and, through exploration, will enable you to be more in harmony with your life's aspirations.

It will help you to establish all the things that are of true value and importance to you. The more balance you seek, the more you will feel in harmony with yourself, at ease and in the flow. All these aspects will impact on the many choices that you make in connection with your wellbeing. Achieving balance will provide you with sustainable high levels of motivation. This, in turn, will help to keep you on track in sustaining this low-GI Plan effortlessly, as part of your positive lifestyle change, beyond these initial 10 days.

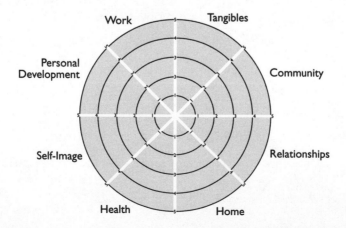

Make your own personal Wheel of Fortune based around the areas shown in the picture, opposite. If some of these areas are not really important to you, leave them out or replace them with others that are more meaningful to you. To help you we have provided an imaginary scale of 1 to 5. Plot your score as you ask yourself the questions shown: 1 represents little to no satisfaction in that particular area of your life and 5 means you are a happy chappy!

The Wheel of Fortune enables you to see, at a glance, where you currently score high or low in your life. Think of it as a snapshot in time. Notice how satisfied you feel with what this has revealed. If your particular wheel is uneven and seemingly all over the place, don't despair – this is a positive thing. It is showing you where changes need to happen. Spend some quality time working through the different areas and scoring yourself honestly. The lower scores indicate where you may wish to make some changes in order to rebalance your life.

Ask yourself these questions and plot your score between 1 and 5.

❑ **Self-Image**: If you could be the kind of person you want to be, what five qualities would you need? How many of these do you already have? Score yourself accordingly.

❑ **Tangibles**: What material things would you like to own? How close to owning these are you today on a scale of 1 to 5?

❑ **Home**: What is your ideal living environment? How near are you to achieving this on a scale of 1 to 5?

❑ **Health:** What is your goal for health, fitness, sports and anything to do with your body? Using the scale, how close are you to reaching this?

❑ **Relationships:** What type of relationships would you like to have with friends, family and others? Using the scale, how close are you to doing so? What would you need to do differently?

❑ **Work:** What impact would you like your efforts to have on your professional or vocational situation? Using the scale, how close are you to achieving this? What changes would you want to make?

❑ **Personal Development:** What would you like to create in the arena of individual learning, travel, reading or similar activities? Where on the scale do you rate yourself now?

❑ **Community:** What is your vision for your local community? What impact have you made in achieving this so far, on a scale of 1 to 5? What would you choose to do more or less of?

For example, if you have scored an honest 2 in health, ask yourself what you must do to get that up to at least a 4 or 5. How would you know that you have achieved this? What would you **see**, **hear** and **feel**? Set yourself some measurable and specific outcomes. For example, saying you'd feel more energetic isn't specific enough. But the following are:

❑ I am working out at the gym for 45 minutes, four times a week.

❑ I am walking 10,000 steps a day (using a step counter to record your steps).

❑ I am riding my bike three times a week for a minimum of one hour.

Choose up to three realistic, tangible and achievable small goals for each area in which you wish to improve your score. Alternatively you could choose to work on a couple only, within a given time frame.

For each of the sections in your personal Wheel of Fortune, add pictures, symbols and/or words to your DreamBoard™ as a visible reminder of what you are focusing on and working towards.

Setting goals means your days will be driven by your life's mission rather than dictated by your moods.

Step 2: Select Your Menu (day 10)

Your meal plan is based on a daily target of 17 GiPs, split on average as follows:

Breakfast:	4 GiPs
Mid-morning booster:	2 GiPs
Lunch:	5 GiPs
Mid-afternoon pick-me-up:	1 GiP
Dinner:	4 GiPs
Evening comforter:	1 GiP

You don't need to count the GiPs; it's all been done for you.

You can make your own menus using the GiP tables so long as you keep to these amounts.

You can have unlimited amounts of GiP-free veg (see table, page 293), including as much as you like of the GiP-free recipes (page 199).

For drinks throughout the day: 200 ml (⅓ pint) skimmed or semi-skimmed milk, unlimited herbal teas, unsweetened tea and coffee, sugar-free drinks, water.

For lunch: These suggestions are low GI, filling and varied. You will be preparing most the previous evening. If some days you can't be bothered, you can opt for a low- or medium-GI sandwich from Marks & Spencer's 'Count on Us' range (check labels), a Sainsbury's GI-tested sandwich (see tables, page 281) or a tailor-made sandwich from a sandwich bar using our suggested low-GI ingredients (see *Getting Ready for Day One*, page 43). You are more likely to get results with the suggested lunches here.

The evening comforter is optional. If you don't like evening snacks, have the comforter at any other time of the day.

Men — have an extra 3 GiPs each day. Check out the tables at the back for GiP values of everyday foods.

Breakfast

Any 4-GiP cereal of your choice (see tables, page 283).
OR
1 glass of unsweetened fruit juice (150 ml).
1 slice multigrain bread, toasted, with a scraping of half-fat
    unsaturated or low-fat spread.
1 tsp reduced-sugar jam.

Mid-morning booster

10 cashew nuts.
OR
4 dried apricots.

Lunch

Sardines on toast: 4 canned sardines (in brine or tomato sauce).
2 slices Burgen soya and linseed toast.
1 satsuma or 1 kiwi fruit.
OR
Egg and tomato roll: Warburtons All In One Roll, scraping of
   low-fat spread, one sliced boiled egg, sliced tomato,
   crispy lettuce and seasoning.
1 apple and 1 firm pear.

Mid-afternoon pick-me-up

1 diet yoghurt.
OR
Olive and Cucumber Snack Box (throw together 10 black or
   green olives, cucumber sticks, and any combination of the
   following: celery sticks, radishes, pickled onions, gherkins,
   water chestnuts)
1 satsuma.

Dinner

These dinner choices are super-speedy. The first looks like a
selection from a Greek meze or Mexican tapas bar, yet this
choice, and even the pan-fried turkey, can be ready in about
15 minutes.

Crispy Tortilla Chips (see recipe, page 208).

Spicy Baked Beans (see recipe, page 222), served hot or cold.

Aubergine Dip (see recipe, Creamed Aubergine with Garlic, page 221).

Mixed Pepper Salsa (see recipe, page 211) and/or Speedy Salsa Sauce (see recipe, page 209).

Optional extra for hungry days: Lemony Chestnut Mushrooms (see recipe, page 216), or any salad or GiP-free vegetables of your choice.

GiP-free Strawberry and Mint Crush (see recipe, page 274).

This selection of delights takes less than 5 minutes for each dish, although the aubergine takes a couple of minutes longer. You can prepare the beans and salsa while the tortilla chips and aubergine are cooking.

OR

Pan-fried Turkey Breasts with Cajun Spice and Tarragon (see recipe, page 232).

½ large can of chilli beans.

Side salad: mixed salad leaves, celery, cucumber, and tomato wedges flavoured with coarse-grain mustard and balsamic vinegar or fat-free dressing.

Strawberry and Mint Crush (see recipe, page 274).

Prepare the salad while the turkey is cooking.
All done in about 15 minutes!

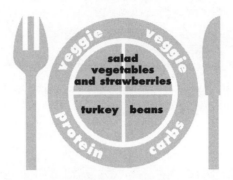

My GI Tip: Any addition of a low-GI food will lower the
Glycaemic Index of the meal – so add chilli beans to
your bolognaise sauce for a lower-GI meal.

MARY MCDERMOTT RD, REGISTERED DIETITIAN

Evening comforter (optional)

Diet hot chocolate made up from a sachet with water or
skimmed milk.

OR

1 rich tea biscuit with a hot drink using milk from allowance.

Step 3: Get GiP Fit (day 10)

Remember, you may combine these into one 20-minute burst
if you prefer.

a) Fitness Burst 1: 10 mins in the morning or at lunchtime

Congratulations! This is the last day of your 10-day plan and
already you'll be feeling the benefits of your efforts. Celebrate

by choosing your favourite dance track for your first 10-minute fitness burst and feel great for the rest of the day.

b) Fitness Burst 2: 10 mins at lunchtime or in the evening
Go cycling for this final 10-minute fitness burst and, again, congratulate yourself on your achievements.

Action point

Think about times when you are standing about, such as talking on the telephone, and do simple stretches such as calf raises: lift your heels off the floor and then lower them again. Repeat as often as feels comfortable.

Step 4: Time in, time out (day 10)

Your two-minute springboard!

Go to the *Practical Tools* section (page 354) and list your three achievements for today. You now have a long list of uplifting successes to refer to whenever you feel you need a confidence boost.

Tiffin Box

Well, now lunch is up to you. Congratulate yourself on having kept as close as you can to this unique 10-day low-GI Diet. Tomorrow is another day. You've created some admirable new habits in terms of eating regularly, eating more fruit and veg, and generally keeping to a healthier lifestyle. Now it's up to you to see what tomorrow and the future in general is going to bring. It's Celebration Friday tomorrow, so do enjoy yourself. However, think about where you are now and whether you would like to enjoy even more weight loss, fat loss or inch loss.

This is about healthy lifestyles, not dieting. Now that you have completed your 10 days, you have adopted new healthier habits. You simply need to carry on making those low-GI choices, like filling half your plate with salad or veg, choosing low-GI carbs like pasta, sweet potatoes, lentils, wholegrain breads, and so on. If you like having a target number of GiPs to aim for, then look up page 178 for advice on your Lose-it phase of the Gi Plan. If you prefer to be more relaxed, then simply follow the main principles of the diet; choose some of the recipes (Chapter 8) and keep as close as you can to the GiP rules. It's all there for the taking in *Beyond 10 days* (Chapter 6).

Take a 'Me Moment'

Touch is important for our overall sense of wellbeing. Treat yourself and book a massage, or get someone close to you to oblige.

Power Tips

❑ Contributing selflessly to the wider community can boost your emotional health.

❑ You can control your appetite by controlling your blood sugar. Maintaining slow, steady rises in blood sugar helps reduce appetite.

❏ Physical fitness can be time enjoyed alone or with others. It absorbs you in something other than your problems and, if you choose, joining a club encourages social contact and meeting new friends.

❏ A problem shared is a problem doubled! But halved, when you have a wise friend to turn to.

05

FRIDAY – CELEBRATION DAY!

Welcome to the rest of your life! In 10 days, that's just 10 days out of your whole life, you have managed to achieve something that clearly means a lot to you. Your new choices will set you up for life and, even after this short period of time, may well have become second nature. New habits form just as quickly as the not-so-healthy ones! Measure your waist and weight and record them in the *Practical Tools* section (page 360). Congratulations. Here are some ideas for the reward scheme!

Balloon 1: Treat yourself and a friend/partner/the family to a take-away meal

☐ Have a low-GI snack before you visit the place.

☐ Whatever you choose, picturing your VVPC plate can help to keep even this indulgence in balance.

☐ Go for lower-calorie choices such as tandoori chicken, stir-fried vegetables, steamed rice, chicken tikka, chargrilled kebabs, grilled meat and fish, and piles of salad.

Balloon 2: Share it with friends

❑ Go dancing at a club or local dance night. Let your hair down and continue to burn off the calories without even realising it.

❑ Enjoy a celebration glass of bubbly. Have up to three units of alcohol, ideally with food.

❑ Have some friends round to join in the celebrations. You can combine this with a take-away and a glass of something and share with them how you did what you did. Perhaps it'll motivate them, too?

Balloon 3: Your personal reward

❑ Book in for a special beauty treatment day. Guys, these exist for you, too. (They're often called pampering exclusively for men!)

❑ Go window shopping and, if you have time, try on some clothes that will show off your new figure. If you have the money, treat yourself – after all, you deserve it!

❑ Treat yourself to something you've often longed to do, like go to the theatre, book a weekend away or just huddle on the sofa with a good video and a friend.

06

BEYOND 10 DAYS

The best way to carry on with your GI healthier, fitter lifestyle is to take on board the practical and punchy tips in the original *Gi Plan*, available from most bookshops. Specific chapters to get stuck into include *Snack Attack, Hasty and Tasty – Meal and Menu Ideas*, and *Eating Out the GiP Way*.

> My GI Tip: There is research to show that people who naturally eat a lower-GI diet appear to be at a lower risk of developing conditions such as type 2 diabetes and heart disease. Regular low-GI eating can help 'apple-shaped' people reduce the unhealthy fat they carry around their abdomen.
>
> DR MARGARET ASHWELL OBE, CONSULTANT NUTRITION SCIENTIST

So, you've now had a taste of low-GI eating and the benefits it brings to your energy levels. What are you going to do now? Is this a crossroads? Are you absolutely convinced that you want to carry on? Chances are, you've got the low-GI bug by now, and carrying on is the only option for you as you are now committed to enjoying a new healthier lifestyle. You will have lost some weight if you have kept to the plan. This is the first phase of the Gi Plan, called the *Start-it Phase*. The original *Gi Plan* book (details under *Further Support & Information*, page 367) will give you extensive information on the different phases of the diet, but for now here is a concise version to help you achieve sustainable results.

If you like the GiP-counting system, then this bit's for you…

The GiP phases

Start-it ⇒ Lose-it ⇒ Keep-it

The Gi Plan is split into three phases. Each has been carefully designed to guide you to your desired goal in an optimum way. It is important that you follow the instructions below to reach your target weight and stay there.

Start-it Phase

The Start-it Phase is designed to kick-start your weight loss, but is only appropriate for around the first two weeks. This has been your 10-day plan. During this phase you are likely to lose weight reasonably quickly.

Lose-it Phase

The second phase, Lose-it, allows you more daily GiPs. This is designed to help you eat more and lose weight more steadily and sensibly. The British Dietetic Association recommends that the ideal rate of weight loss is around 0.5–1 kg (1–2 lbs) per week.

The key to long-term weight loss: lose
0.5–1 kg (1–2 lbs) per week and no more!

If you go for fewer GiPs, you'll probably lose weight more quickly. But research shows that trying to lose weight too quickly is not effective in keeping the weight off permanently. You are more likely to put the weight back on, as with many other diets. So keep it slow and steady, especially since losing weight too quickly can be harmful in the long term.

Having more GiPs during the Lose-it Phase means you can eat more. Not only does this feel fab, it helps you to avoid hunger too. Feeling full and including more daily GiPs means that this phase fits more easily into your lifestyle.

Keep-it Phase

One you've reached a more desirable weight, the GiP system helps you keep hold of your new lifestyle. You are in charge of how many GiPs you need to keep you slim and fit.

How many GiPs for me?

In general, women are likely to lose an appropriate and steady amount of weight on 20 GiPs per day, and 25 GiPs a day is likely to best suit men. Use the following table to work out your daily GiPs.

	Start-it Phase (2 weeks) GiPs per day	Lose-it Phase (to target) GiPs per day	Keep-it Phase (staying on target) GiPs per day
Women	17	20	23 or more
Men	20–22	22–25	28 or more

And as for alcohol…for weight management we recommend no more than 7 units of alcohol per week, with two to three alcohol-free days. So, in the Lose-it Phase, enjoy an extra 4 units (with a maximum of 7 units per week) and in the Keep-it Phase you can increase this to a maximum of about 14–21 units per week, as recommended by health organisations.

The tables on page 281 will open up a wide range of choices to help you keep to your daily GiPs target. Remember also the tempting recipes (Chapter 8), which have all been GiP calculated for you.

When you are ready to slide into the Lose-it Phase, remind yourself of the GiP rules (Chapter 1) so that you continue to get results.

If you just want to carry on with healthier low-GI eating, then this bit's for you...

If you don't like worrying about portion sizes, and simply want to enjoy a healthier lifestyle rather than lose weight, then GI is for you. Simply take on board the GI tips and include one low-GI carb at every meal. For example, choose muesli or multigrain bread for breakfast, pasta for lunch and low-GI carbs like bulgur wheat, whole new potatoes in their skins or basmati rice in the evening. Look up the GiP tables (page 281) and choose those low-GI foods that you enjoy, but forget about the counting. Keep it simple and you'll still get results.

Here's a checklist that will help to keep you on track:

❑ Look back at the GiP rules in *GI and the Gi Plan* (Chapter 1) – the only one that would not apply to you is GiP Rule 2.

❑ Remind yourself of the shopping essentials and lunchtime swaps, *Getting Ready for Day 1* (Chapter 3).

❑ Check out the *Top 100 Tips* (Chapter 7). They will provide you with renewed energy to carry on.

❑ Keep monitoring your waist and weight (include body fat measurements, if you have chosen to do this). Continue to record this under *Practical Tools* (Chapter 10).

❑ Consider attending a Gi Plan workshop, details under *Further Support & Information* (page 367).

❑ Check out the website, www.giplan.com for new inspirational tips.

❑ Flick through the original *The Gi Plan* for more hints, tips and sound nutritional guidance.

Always choose the active option

✗ Take the kids to the pictures.

✔ **Take them swimming.**

✗ Go to the pub.

✔ **Play a game of tennis, then pub.**

✗ Sit down for a coffee and chat.

✔ **Get a group of mums/mates, and power walk and chat.**

✔ If applicable, even better, **take baby and pram.**

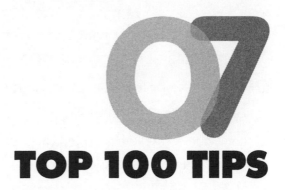

TOP 100 TIPS

Here are 100 great ways to stay slim, fit, healthy and young, split up into 10 categories.

1 Eternal youth

- ❑ Research suggests that thinking young could prolong your age.
- ❑ Perceived lower age indicates optimism, which suggests a reduction in the risk of illness.
- ❑ Building meaningful relationships with friends and family has been shown to reduce ageing.
- ❑ Pets, especially dogs, reduce stress and can keep you youthful for longer.
- ❑ Laughter reduces stress and tension and strengthens the immune system. Laugh a lot!
- ❑ Keep your finances in order. Feeling out of control can increase the risk of ageing.
- ❑ It is said that daily exercise can reduce your 'real' age by years.

❑ Make a list of personal stress busters. For example, walking, dancing, yoga or time spent in good company.

❑ Take up a new interest or hobby – anything that allows you the freedom to switch off.

❑ Let it out! A chat with a trusted chum can work wonders in supporting you and relieving your anxieties.

2 Ten reasons to go on the 10-day Gi diet

❑ Let's face it, diets can get boring. The difference with the 10-day Gi Diet is that it's flexible and fun and it allows you to give a new eating plan a try for just a few days.

❑ There are at least 20 different studies that suggest that if you slow down carbohydrate digestion, you promote satiety signals (feeling of fullness).

❑ When you are on a strict diet, your metabolic rate may fall – and that means you don't burn off fat so quickly. Studies show that the fall in metabolic rate is less on a low-GI diet.

❑ Generally, when you reduce the energy density of foods, you increase the fibre and the feeling of fullness. The GiP system is based on both energy density and GI. A winning combination.

❑ Studies show that you burn more fat after eating low-GI foods.

❏ Fashionable meets science – no other popular diet has 25 years of research behind it.

❏ The GiP system provides you with a counting system that helps you to be in charge of what you eat, and have the flexibility to enjoy your favourite foods.

❏ Lose fat, not muscle – two groups of rats were fed different diets, based on their GI. The study showed that the rats fed low-GI foods could eat more food yet keep to the same weight as the high-GI group. There was 70 per cent more body fat in rats fed the high-GI diet.

❏ You can manage diabetes by eating more low-GI foods as part of your plan.

❏ Glucose 'spikes' stimulate appetite. You can keep your glucose levels steady by focusing on low-GiP carbs.

3 Positively positive

❏ Treat yourself to a consultation with a personal shopper.

❏ Get a new hair style.

❏ Book in for an aromatherapy massage.

❏ Surround yourself with happy people.

❏ Put aside a couple of hours weekly to watch funny DVDs.

❏ Get a makeover.

❏ Set yourself small, achievable goals and feel great when you achieve them.

☐ Look forward to as many things in a day as you can create.

☐ Do a good deed regardless of whether or not there's anything in it for you!

☐ Train yourself to wake up to an immediate happy thought every morning.

4 Physical activity – why bother? Here's why! Regular exercise...

☐ Delays ageing.

☐ Enhances flexibility.

☐ Increases self-esteem.

☐ Acts as a stress buster.

☐ Lessens lower-back pain and helps strengthen the back.

☐ Reduces the symptoms of pre-mentrual syndromes (PMS).

☐ Helps the heart beat stronger.

☐ Helps reduce asthma attacks.

☐ Enhances posture.

☐ Helps improve varicose veins.

5 Ten shopping list essentials

☐ Lower-fat dairy products, e.g. semi-skimmed milk, reduced-fat cheese.

☐ Fresh fruit, canned fruit in juice.

☐ Dried fruit, e.g. apricots.

☐ Vegetables, fresh, frozen and canned.

☐ High-fibre cereals, e.g. original porridge oats (large flake), All Bran, muesli.

☐ Lower-GI bread, e.g. granary, multigrain, tortilla wraps.

☐ Yoghurt, natural, virtually fat-free/diet.

☐ Rice and grains, e.g. brown rice, basmati rice, bulgur wheat, couscous.

☐ Dried or canned beans, any variety.

☐ Pasta, any type.

6 Are you getting enough? (Relaxation!)

☐ Get a good night's sleep on a regular basis.

☐ Free yourself of the guilt concept. If you're not doing anything, it's okay, really!

☐ Doing less and 'being' more can lead to greater success and happiness.

☐ If you fear the competition of 'who's got the fullest diary' among your friends and colleagues, start a new trend of 'who's got the most blank pages'!

☐ Relaxation can mean bigger achievements as it improves your focus and increases your commitment.

❏ Ideally, aim for at least a few minutes' relaxation each day, a few hours each week, a few days each month.

❏ Think about how you'd like to use this free time and tell your family/partner, so they know to honour it, too.

❏ Choose a lovely tranquil location to walk in.

❏ Choose a time and make a conscious decision to turn off your mobile. Life will go on without you being on the end of the phone!

❏ If you have decided to relax with a glass of wine and chat with your best chum, do that, and that only. Forget multi-tasking; wrestling with the ironing, feeding the dog or cooking the dinner at the same time!

7 Burn off the cals, here's how...

❏ Ironing for half an hour can burn up to 150 calories.

❏ 30 minutes of vacuuming can shed up to 200 calories.

❏ 250 calories can be lost while cleaning the windows – and with all that stretching on your tippy toes, you will tone the arms, thighs, love handles and shoulders, too!

❏ Using the stairs 10 times a day will see another 250 calories melt away, while toning the thighs and bottom.

❏ Check your room temperature. A warm environment slows down the rate at which you burn calories, so reset the thermostat – and save money too!

❑ If gardening is your thing, 30 minutes can burn off around 150 calories.

❑ Cycling is a great incentive for burning calories and an hour on your bike can help you lose around 330.

❑ A brisk walk, so you feel yourself getting slightly out of breath and sweaty, for 15 minutes at a rate of 4 mph, can burn 100 calories, effortlessly.

❑ Your brain becomes more energised when you stand while working or studying. Plug in your standing time at least 5 times a day for 10 minutes, preferably every hour. This could see a further 25 per cent of calories burn away.

❑ Sex burns 400 calories an hour (or 100 calories every 15 minutes).

8 Ten health boosters

❑ More than 70 per cent of the salt you eat is added to your food by the manufacturer, often without you even knowing it.

❑ Men – watch that waist. Men typically carry more fat around their belly. Note that a waist measurement of more than 94 cm/37 in (90 cm/36 in for Asian men) increases your risk of heart disease. If your waist measurement is as high as 100 cm (40 in), it really is time to take some serious action.

❑ Sweet potatoes are an excellent source of the antioxidant beta-carotene, which the body can convert into vitamin A. This vitamin is essential for healthy skin and eyesight.

❏ The GiP diet encourages a variety of foods from all the food groups. If followed, it should contain enough nutrients to meet your daily needs. However, dieters often prefer to take a multivitamin and mineral supplement as well. If you do so, ensure that you choose one that has no more than 100 per cent recommended daily amount (RDA) of nutrients.

❏ The Inuit population's traditional diet was high in animal fat yet it protected them against heart disease. The fat came primarily from cold-water fish, rich in omega-3 fatty acids.

❏ Lacking in concentration? Try starting your day with a high-bran cereal mixed with a handful of raisins. The B vitamins are crucial for transmitting nerve signals.

❏ Trans fats are often found in processed foods, many of which have a high-GI rating. These act just like saturated fats in your body, raising your blood cholesterol and clogging your artery walls, making you more prone to heart problems.

❏ Suffer from fatigue? This could be a sign of low iron levels. Look at labels and select those foods that have been enriched with this mineral. Red meat, dark poultry meat, dark green leafy vegetables, lentils, fortified breakfast cereals and dried apricots are all good iron providers.

❏ Kids behaving badly? Choosing healthy low-GI meals and snacks for children can help to improve their concentration, as well as sustain steady energy levels.

❏ Getting forgetful? There is good research to show that omega-3 fats may play an important role in memory, especially in the elderly.

9 Happy times ahead!

❏ Take pleasure in simple things.

❏ Live your own life, not someone else's.

❏ Adopt an attitude of gratitude. Be thankful for all you have and all you haven't, too!

❏ Don't worry about what hasn't happened. It's a wasteful pastime.

❏ Support those who are less fortunate, when you can.

❏ Let go of anything that's holding you back, such as past mistakes, grudges or similar negative feelings towards others.

❏ Make up your mind to do what you love and love what you do.

❏ There is no failure, only growth through the stumbling.

❏ Increase your flexibility. The person with the greatest flexibility will ultimately control most outcomes.

❏ Trust in the process of life. Believe there's a higher purpose to everything.

10 Ten ways to lower GI

❑ Whenever you have a salad, add an acidic dressing, such as lime juice.

❑ Whenever you have pasta, keep it *al dente* (firm to the bite).

❑ Before you buy a banana, check that it is under-ripe and has a green tipped skin and therefore is low GI.

❑ Whenever you have a jacket potato, add a little low-GI carb such as baked beans.

❑ Remember 'Veggie, Veggie, Protein, Carbs' and picture your plate regularly like this. Fruits count in the veggie section.

❑ Keep your vegetables raw or undercooked.

❑ Have fresh fruit instead of fruit juice.

❑ Add beans or lentils to stews and casseroles.

❑ Experiment with lower-GI carbs such as bulgur wheat, quinoa, brown rice and couscous.

❑ Here's a golden rule: generally, the more processing the food industry does, the less processing your gut has to do. Keep it whole and natural so your gut has to do more work.

08

THE RECIPES

These recipes have been planned with health in mind. They are low fat and incorporate a range of low-GI carbs. Each has been Gipped using the tables at the back of the book, so all you need to do is to slot them into your daily menus, before, during and after your 10-day plan. The best news is that almost all of them can be on the table in about 20 minutes. And you don't need to be a super-chef to be able to boil some pasta and throw in a can of tomatoes and some herbs. They are so simple that you might surprise yourself with what you can create by just adding different ingredients to a pan.

About the recipes

All the recipes have been tested using metric measures, but if you prefer old-fashioned imperial, then simply go to page 275 for a conversion list. You will also see temperature conversions for gas and electric cookers on this page.

Since we don't know whether you only cook for yourself or you want to cook healthy family meals, we have made these recipes flexible enough for both. Most of the recipes in this section have been created for one person, but if you want to serve four people, then simply adjust the quantities. Note that some cooking times may increase when you increase the amount of ingredients.

You can use GiP-free veg, flavourings and herbs in any quantities you like, so if you prefer more or less of any of these ingredients, feel free to adjust. In some cases a recipe for one may need ⅓ of a pepper – if you are cooking for four, one pepper would be fine. Think about what's practical for you. Similarly, instead of doubling up '4 tbsp chopped coriander leaves and stems' just throw in a couple of handfuls. Allowing yourself such flexibility increases your cooking confidence. It's also much more fun and liberating if you're not tied down to specific quantities. You can do this with all GiP-free ingredients.

You may find that a recipe demands spices, such as turmeric or cumin seeds. If you like these flavours buying the ingredients will pay off, as there are a few recipes that use the same basic ingredients.

There are around 70 recipes in this section, and about a quarter of them are GiP-free, but if you want more, then you can always refer to the original *Gi Plan* book which is available from most bookstores.

Alternatives

Here are some tips on alternatives to the ingredients in the recipes:

❏ You can use any herbs you like, in any amounts. Fresh herbs will give you a much more authentic and aromatic flavour, but you can substitute a good pinch of dried herbs if you like.

❏ Add any of the free flavourings from the free flavourings list.

❏ You can double up or halve recipes as necessary.

❏ Sometimes there will be suggested accompaniments, and you can choose to use these or not.

❏ Substitute shallots, red onion or spring onion for ordinary onions. Or the other way around!

❏ The recipes recommend that you use an olive oil spray. These are available in supermarkets, though you may prefer to make your own from scratch. Simply mix one part olive oil to seven parts of water and pour into a pump-spray bottle, which you can buy from good kitchenware stores. When using a spray oil, it's best to heat the pan before adding oil. Always use a non-stick pan. Add one or two tbsp hot water if food begins to stick to the bottom of the pan (no need to add any extra oil). Even by putting oil into a pump-spray bottle without added water you're likely to use less.

Want short cuts?

❏ Use passata or chopped canned tomatoes instead of fresh.

❏ Try canned lentils instead of dried.

❑ Choose frozen vegetables instead of fresh.

❑ Go for cut carrot batons or cherry tomatoes, for quick and convenient salads and snacks.

❑ For chicken recipes, you could buy some pre-cooked chicken from the supermarket. Remember to check the 'best-by' date and store as recommended.

❑ Or you could freeze strips of chicken and defrost when you're ready to create some of the chicken dishes.

❑ Some of the recipes and menu plans use our eat-now-eat-later strategy. So you could prepare roasted vegetables one evening and use the leftovers for, say, a roasted vegetable and ricotta cheese sandwich the next day.

❑ Try making a large pot of soup so that it lasts you for more than one serving.

❑ Use a food processor to chop vegetables.

❑ Boil a load of pasta and freeze in individual portions (115 g per serving), then defrost and use as required.

❑ Dishes like Red Lentil Dahl with Lime and Coriander and Aromatic Basmati Rice can easily be frozen, so you could make enough for more than one serving and freeze the rest.

❑ Make the Beefier Burgers and freeze them raw. Then all you need to do is thaw and grill.

Lentils and beans

These recipes use canned beans and lentils for ease of cooking and to save time. Standard cans are around the same size, so the recipes simply state whether you need a large can, half a can or a small can.

Recipe list

SOUPS, STARTERS AND SIDES

Tomato Soup with Crunchy Onions and Green Pepper 'Croutons'

---

0 GiPs per serving

GiP-free speedy recipe

This is so simple to make, you'll feel like you're cheating in the kitchen, and your friends need never know you haven't spent ages skinning, de-seeding, chopping and sieving the tomatoes. Passata (sieved tomatoes) can be bought in jars or cartons and should be a staple in any (cheating) cook's cupboard. Keep the coriander and onions crunchy and undercooked, as this adds more texture. For a vegetarian option, use vegetable rather than chicken stock. Ready in about 10 minutes.

Serves 2

Olive oil spray
1 onion, roughly chopped
2 tsp crushed garlic from a jar
300 ml passata (sieved tomatoes)
150 ml chicken stock (made up from ½ stock cube and 150 ml boiling water)
4 tbsp roughly chopped coriander leaves and stems
2 tbsp roughly chopped basil leaves
2 spring onions, sliced
⅓ green pepper, diced into small squares
Freshly ground black pepper to taste
Few drops of chilli sauce (optional)

1. Preheat the grill to medium and line a grill pan with foil. Heat a non-stick pan, add 10 sprays of oil and fry the onion and garlic over a medium heat for a few seconds. Add a couple of tablespoons of hot water to prevent the onions from burning.
2. Put the passata, chicken stock, herbs, spring onions and seasoning into the pan and bring to the boil.
3. Lower the heat and simmer for about 5 minutes. Meanwhile, grill the peppers under a moderately hot grill till charred.
4. Adjust the seasoning, add chilli sauce (if using) and serve hot, garnished with the grilled pepper 'croutons'.

Nutrition Nuggets: This is GiP-free so if you're really hungry, you can have the whole amount for yourself. There's no need to add salt as you get plenty from the stock cube. The recipe creatively substitutes the carbs and calories from standard bread croutons with vitamin C-rich and low-GI green peppers. Great for a night-time supper or snack on a cold winter's evening.

Rustic Red Lentil and Basil Soup

1 GiP per serving

Some lentils need presoaking or they may take a while to cook, but red lentils are one of the speediest lentils to prepare. You can use any fresh herbs instead of the basil if you prefer. Fresh coriander and parsley work particularly well.

If you are really pushed for time use a pressure cooker at step 2 and follow the manufacturer's instructions.

Serves 2

Olive oil spray
½ onion, chopped
1 tsp crushed garlic
½ can chopped tomatoes
125 g red lentils, washed
300 ml vegetable stock (made from 1 stock cube and 300 ml boiling water)
Generous handful of basil leaves
¼ tsp dried parsley
Coarse black pepper

1. Heat a non-stick pan and add 10 sprays of oil. Gently stir-fry the onion and garlic to soften, adding a couple of tablespoons of hot water if the mixture begins to stick to the bottom.
2. Add the tomatoes, lentils and 300 ml boiling water. Cover and simmer till cooked (about 10–15 minutes).
3. Add the stock, whole basil leaves, parsley and black pepper. Heat through for about a minute and serve.

Nutrition Nuggets: In this wholesome recipe, the lentils are cooked but not puréed. This helps to preserve a lower GI.

Farmhouse Barley and Lentil Broth

2 GiPs per serving

Barley is one of the lowest-GI grains and it works particularly well in a soup. If you have a pressure cooker, then follow the manufacturer's instructions for cooking times. Otherwise, simply allow this to cook slowly for 1–1½ hours. This recipe makes a hearty family meal, or you can simply cut down on the ingredients to suit your required number of servings.

Serves 6

125 g pearl barley
125 g mixed lentils
2 litres vegetable stock (fresh or made with 3 stock cubes and
    2 litres boiling water)
Olive oil spray
1 onion, finely chopped
1 large carrot, sliced
6 courgettes, diced
150 g spinach, chopped
2 tsp dried mixed herbs

1. Cook the barley with the lentils in 600 ml of hot stock either in a pressure cooker or in a pan, as above.
2. Heat a large non-stick pan and add 10 sprays of oil. Add the onion and carrots and stir-fry over a low heat till soft. Add some hot water if the mixture begins to stick to the bottom.
3. Add the courgettes and spinach and stir-fry for a few minutes. Stir in the cooked barley and lentil mixture with

the remaining vegetable stock. Add the herbs and season to taste. (Add more water as required if you prefer it to be thinner.)

Nutrition Nuggets: This broth combines the very best of low-GI carbohydrates with colourful vegetables to provide a healthy range of nutrients.

Chilled Gazpacho

0 GiPs per serving

This GiP-free recipe is great for warm summer evenings or as a mid-afternoon pick-me-up snack. If you can, it's a good idea to put all the ingredients in the fridge before you start preparing this dish. Then it is ready to eat as soon as you've whizzed it up in a food processor or blender.

Serves 1

4 tomatoes
½ red pepper, chopped
1 tsp crushed garlic
½ red onion, chopped
1 tbsp tomato purée
2 tsp red wine vinegar
Handful of basil leaves, chopped
Salt and ground black pepper
Dash of Worcester sauce
Salt and pepper

To serve:

Whole basil leaves

¼ red onion, sliced

1. Simply blitz all these ingredients together in a food processor or blender, and chill in the refrigerator.
2. Serve garnished with fresh basil leaves and chopped red onion.

Nutrition Nuggets: Vegetables such as tomatoes provide potassium, an important mineral that helps to regulate blood pressure.

Hot and Sour Soup

0 GiPs per serving

This quick-and-easy soup is a great winter warmer when you fancy something light yet satisfying and GiP-free. However, you can also transform it into a more satisfying main meal soup. To do this, swirl in 2 beaten eggs at Step 3 instead of the egg white. Then add any of your favourite vegetables. Fennel, French beans, mangetout, beansprouts and sweetcorn go particularly well. Remember to add the GiPs from the egg (3 GiPs) and/or the sweetcorn (3 tbsp count as 2.5 GiPs).

Serves 1

Olive oil spray

2 baby leeks or large spring onions, sliced

½ tsp crushed ginger

450 ml chicken or vegetable stock (made with 1 stock cube
    crumbled into 450 ml boiling water)
Generous handful of pak choi or baby spinach
1 tsp Thai fish sauce, or to taste
1 tbsp soy sauce
2 tsp wine vinegar
15 g coriander leaves and stems, chopped roughly
To serve:
1 egg white
Chilli sauce or coarse black pepper, as desired
1 lemon slice, washed (unpeeled)

1. Heat a non-stick pan and add 10 sprays of oil. Stir-fry the baby leeks and crushed ginger for about 1 minute, adding a couple of tablespoons of hot water if the leeks begin to stick to the bottom.

2. Add all the remaining ingredients and cook for about 3–4 minutes, until the leeks are tender.

3. Swirl the egg white into the pan while stirring, to create a marbled effect as it cooks. Cover the pan with a lid for about a minute to allow the egg to set.

4. Add chilli sauce or pepper, throw in the fresh lemon slice and serve.

Cheat's Whole Lentil and Coriander Soup

I GiP per serving

This recipe uses canned green lentils as a speedy 10-minute shortcut for a filling soup. If you like, you can use this as an eat-now-eat-later recipe. Simply cook the whole can, double up the other ingredients and then use the remaining half of the soup to make Green Lentil Dahl (see recipe, page 259).

Serves I

Olive oil spray
½ onion, finely chopped
I tsp crushed garlic
100 ml passata
150 ml vegetable stock (made using fresh vegetable stock, vegetable bouillon or ½ stock cube in 150 ml boiling water)
½ can green lentils, drained
Generous handful of coriander leaves and stems, chopped

1. Heat a non-stick pan, and add 10 sprays of oil, add the onions and garlic. Stir-fry for about 5–8 minutes, till soft.
2. Add the tomatoes, stock and lentils, and cook for a few minutes to heat through.
3. Stir in the coriander and serve hot.

Nutrition Nuggets: Lentils are a fantastic low-GI carbohydrate. But getting the pressure cooker out to cook them isn't always very appealing. Using canned lentils, as in this recipe, is as healthy but less time-consuming. Add a drizzle of lemon juice or a few drops of chilli sauce if you want to give this dish some extra zing.

Warming Marrow and Leek Soup

0 GiPs per serving

Serves 1

*300 ml vegetable stock (made using ½ stock cube in 300 ml
    boiling water)*
200 g marrow, chopped
¼ red pepper, diced
1 leek, sliced
Pinch of dried parsley
Coarse black pepper

1. Heat the stock in a pan and add the vegetables with a
    large pinch of dried parsley.
2. Cook through and add pepper to taste.

Crispy Tortilla Chips

3 GiPs per serving

Make your own crispy wedges at home with tortilla wrap and
your favourite seasoning. If you prefer, cut the wrap into
smaller wedges so it looks like you have more! Use 5 sprays of
oil before adding the seasoning if you like. If you enjoy them
experiment with your own flavourings, like salt and vinegar.

Serves 1

1 tortilla wrap
Flavouring of your choice. Choose any combination of the following:
    Sprinkle of ground cumin

Pinch of salt
Ground black pepper
Sprinkle of red chilli powder
Sprinkle of curry powder

1. Preheat the oven to 200°C. Cut the tortilla wrap into 8 wedges.
2. Sprinkle with your desired seasoning and bake on a baking tray for 2–3 minutes.

Nutrition Nuggets: Bought tortilla chips are generally high in fat, salt and additives. This home-made version has virtually no added fat and is a great accompaniment to dishes such as *Creamed Aubergine with Garlic* or *Speedy Salsa Sauce*.

Speedy Salsa Sauce

0 GiPs per serving

Serves 1

Olive oil spray
½ tsp crushed garlic
½ small onion, finely chopped
¼ red pepper, finely chopped
⅓ can chopped tomatoes
Good pinch of red chilli powder

1. Heat 5 sprays of oil in a non-stick frying pan and add the garlic, onion and red pepper.
2. Add the chopped tomatoes with some of the tomato

juice from the can and flavour with a good pinch of red chilli powder.

3. Simmer for about 3–5 minutes, adding more tomato juice if desired. Serve chilled.

Nutrition Nuggets: Bought sauces may contain additives and other processing ingredients. This recipe offers a simple but possibly more natural way to have all the tangy Mexican flavours yet know exactly what you're eating. Use fresh chopped tomatoes and tomato juice if you prefer.

Stir-fried Noodles with Crispy Vegetables

2 GiPs per serving

You could have this as a main meal – just add a tossed side salad.

Serves 1

50 g thread egg noodles or instant noodles
Olive oil spray
4 spring onions, sliced
½ tsp crushed garlic
½ tsp crushed ginger
1 green chilli, deseeded and chopped (optional)
Generous handful of pak choi (Chinese leaves)
Generous handful of beansprouts
½ can baby sweetcorn, drained
½ can water chestnuts, drained and sliced
½ can bamboo shoots, drained

Good pinch of Chinese five-spice powder
Good pinch of dried basil
1 tbsp soy sauce
Coarse black pepper

1. Cook the noodles in hot water following instructions on the packet. Drain and keep warm.
2. Heat a non-stick wok or large frying pan and add 10 sprays of oil. Stir-fry the onions, garlic and ginger for about ½ a minute.
3. Add all the other ingredients and stir-fry for a few minutes until the vegetables are lightly cooked, but not soft.
4. Stir in the cooked noodles and heat thoroughly. Adjust the seasoning and serve.

Nutrition Nuggets: Throw in as many GiP-free vegetables (see tables, page 293) as you like. It creates a larger portion size and fills you up more.

Mixed Pepper Salsa

0 GiPs per serving

No GiPs means nothing on your hips!

A speedy snack or side dish that is refreshing and nutritious. A piquant accompaniment to a hot curry.

Serves 1

½ red pepper, diced
½ yellow pepper, diced

15 g flat-leaf parsley, chopped
Juice from ½ fresh lime
½ red onion, chopped
Coarse black pepper

1. Simply mix all the ingredients together and serve chilled.

Nutrition Nuggets: Adding this dish to any of your meals will help to fill the veggie portion of the VVPC (veggie veggie protein carbs) plate. For more on this, see Chapter 1.

Tomato and Mustard Seed Salad

0 GiPs per serving

Serves 1

10 cherry tomatoes, halved
1 tsp coarse-grain mustard
Handful of fresh parsley, chopped
1–2 tbsp balsamic vinegar

1. Simply mix all the ingredients together and season as desired.

Nutrition Nuggets: This is a great GiP-free accompaniment to any meal and counts as one of your five-a-day fruit and veg target.

Speedy Cucumber and Mint Raita

I GiP per serving

Use as much of the coriander leaves as you like, and include the crunchy coriander stems, which add a delightful texture to this refreshing accompaniment.

Serves I

150 ml low-fat natural yoghurt
1–2 tsp cumin seeds, as desired
1 tsp mint sauce
2 tbsp freshly chopped coriander leaves and stems
Coarse black pepper
Pinch of red chilli powder (optional)
5-cm piece of cucumber, chopped finely or grated and drained

1. Mix together all the ingredients except the cucumber. Chill in the refrigerator until needed.
2. Stir in the cucumber just before serving.

Nutrition Nuggets: It may surprise you to know that this amount of cucumber contributes one to your five-a-day fruit and veg target.

Caramelised Carrots

0.5 GiPs per serving

Serves I

1 large carrot, peeled and cut into thick diagonal slices
1 tsp dried parsley

Olive oil spray
1 tbsp soy sauce

1. Boil the carrots in the minimum of unsalted hot water in a covered saucepan until just cooked.
2. Drain the cooking water (you can use this for boiling other vegetables or for gravy). Reheat the pan and add the other ingredients to the cooked carrots. Sauté over a high heat until the carrots are lightly charred.
3. Season to taste and add a little more soy sauce to the hot pan if you want to serve the carrots from the pan while still sizzling.

Nutrition Nuggets: Caramelised vegetables usually contain sugar, but this recipe uses a sugar-free method of charring the carrots. The soy sauce adds a nutty flavour and tempting sizzling sounds.

Roasted Sweet Potato Slices

3 GiPs per serving

All you have to do here is peel this unusual vegetable, slice it, throw it into a tray and wait just over 10 minutes for it to cook. Add some chilli sauce if you prefer a mixture of sweet and hot flavours.

Serves 1

Olive oil spray
1 sweet potato, peeled and sliced
Generous pinch of dried mixed herbs

1–2 tbsp Worcester sauce, as desired
Salt and pepper

1. Preheat the oven to 200°C and line an oven tray with foil.
2. Add 5 sprays of oil and lay the sweet potato slices in one layer.
3. Flavour with the herbs, Worcester sauce and seasoning and add another 5 sprays of oil on top.
4. Make a parcel with the foil and bake for about 10–12 minutes till tender.

Nutrition Nuggets: A great alternative to classic potatoes. They offer a lower GI and contain the antioxidant beta-carotene.

Simple Bulgur Wheat

2 GiPs per serving

You really do need to try cooking bulgur wheat before you make your assessment of it. It's not a traditional favourite, but when you start cooking and flavouring it, you may be surprised by its interesting taste and texture.

Serves 1

50 g bulgur wheat
300 ml vegetable stock (made up using fresh stock, vegetable bouillon or ½ stock cube in 300 ml hot water)
3 tbsp freshly chopped parsley or mint
Ground black pepper, to taste

1. Simply put all the ingredients together and cook over a
    moderate heat in a covered pan for about 10–15 minutes
    until all the water is absorbed and the wheat is tender.
    Add pepper to taste.

Nutrition Nuggets: Bulgur wheat has a much lower GI than
rice and couscous. Use it often.

Lemony Chestnut Mushrooms

0 GiPs per serving

These whole chestnut mushrooms are quickly sautéed in a
mixture of lemon thyme and fresh parsley. Delicious also as a
light snack. If you can't be bothered with pots and pans, just
cook the whole thing in the microwave for about 2–3 minutes.

Serves 1

Olive oil spray
¼ onion, finely diced
1 tsp crushed garlic
125 g whole chestnut mushrooms, washed
Few sprigs of fresh lemon thyme (no stalks)
2–3 tbsp lemon juice
2 tbsp chopped parsley

1. Heat a non-stick frying pan and add 10 sprays of oil.
    Quickly sauté the onion and garlic in the oil, adding
    2–3 tbsp of hot water if the onions begin to stick to the
    bottom.

2. Stir in the lemon thyme, lemon juice, and parsley. Cook for about 3 minutes.
3. Add the mushrooms and stir-fry until just tender, around 5 minutes. Serve hot.

Nutrition Nuggets: A great GiP-free addition to any meal.

Roasted Mediterranean Vegetables

0 GiPs per serving

A generous portion size.

Serves 1

1 red pepper, chopped roughly

1 green pepper, chopped roughly

1–2 garlic cloves, peeled and left whole

2 courgettes, sliced

1 small aubergine, chopped

1 red onion, peeled and chopped into large petals

½ tsp dried basil

Few sprigs of rosemary

Salt and pepper

Olive oil spray

1. Preheat the oven to 190°C. Lightly grease an ovenproof dish and warm this in the oven until hot (about 5 minutes).
2. Put all the ingredients into the warmed dish, mix well and season. Add 10 sprays of oil. Roast in the oven for about 20 minutes till cooked but not mushy.

Nutrition Nuggets: Add some low-GI pulses, such as cooked cannellini or borlotti beans, or some marinated tofu, to transform this dish into a tasty vegetarian main course. (Remember to add the GiPs from the other ingredients.) You get three of your 5-a-day fruit and veg from the dish.

Stir-fried Crunchy Vegetables

0 GiPs per serving

This is one of those recipes that you can conjure up in minutes with any frozen, fresh or leftover vegetables. It makes a delicious GiP-free accompaniment to any meal. If you're adjusting quantities to serve four, you can use 2 tsp each of garlic and ginger as this will provide plenty of flavour.

Serves 1

Olive oil spray
1 tsp crushed garlic
1 tsp crushed ginger
½ red pepper, diced
½ green pepper, diced
100 g French beans
100 g mushrooms, sliced
2 spring onions, sliced diagonally
Salt or soy sauce, to taste
Freshly ground black pepper

1. Heat a non-stick wok or pan and add 10 sprays of oil. Stir-fry the garlic, ginger, peppers and French beans until tender. Add 2–3 tbsp of hot water if the mixture begins to stick to the bottom.

2. Stir in the mushrooms and spring onions and cook over a high heat for about 2 minutes. Add the seasoning and serve hot.

Nutrition Nuggets: Keep the vegetables as crunchy as you can – this helps slow down digestion and preserves the nutrients. Try a reduced-salt soy sauce.

Chargrilled Courgette Ribbons

0 GiPs per serving

This speedy dish makes an unusual starter, or an accompaniment to a main meal, or an evening comforter when you feel like a GiP-free but warming snack.

Serves 1

1 courgette, topped and tailed
½ lemon
1 tbsp soy sauce
Good pinch of dried oregano
Good pinch of cumin seeds
Ground black pepper
Olive oil spray

To serve:
Handful of watercress or crispy salad leaves
Good pinch of sesame seeds

1. Preheat the grill to high and line a grill pan with foil. Slice the courgette into ribbons using a Y-shaped vegetable peeler.

2. Lay the courgette ribbons on to the foil. Wash the outside of the lemon and cut into thin slices.
3. Flavour the courgettes with the soy sauce, oregano, cumin seeds and black pepper. Add 5 sprays of oil.
4. Lay the lemon slices around the courgettes and grill for 4–5 minutes till the courgettes are cooked and slightly crispy and browned at the edges.
5. Serve with grilled lemon slices on a bed of watercress or salad leaves, sprinkled with a few sesame seeds.

Nutrition Nuggets: A great dish for filling one of the veggie quarters of your plate (see veggie veggie protein carb plate model, *GI and the Gi Plan*, Chapter 1)

Marmalade Chutney

1 GiP per serving

Serves 1

2 tsp reduced-sugar marmalade
Red chilli powder, to taste
¼ tsp ground cumin seeds
¼ red onion, finely chopped

1. Mix all the ingredients together, add the chilli to taste and serve.

Creamed Aubergine with Garlic

0 GiPs per serving

This is one of the most versatile, GiP-free recipes. You can serve it warm on toast, wrapped in a tortilla, with chapattis and raita, GiP-free as a warming snack, or even cold in a sandwich, as a dip or pâté. If you want it to look special, you can serve the creamed aubergine in the whole aubergine shell – impressive for entertaining.

Serves 1–2

1 aubergine, washed
2 cloves fresh garlic, sliced
Lemon juice, to taste
A little salt, to taste
Good pinch of ground turmeric
1 spring onion, green stems only, sliced
Coarse black pepper
Good pinch of red chilli powder, optional
Few sprigs of coriander leaves

1. Make thick slits into the aubergine with a knife and pierce the garlic slices into the slits. Cook in the microwave for 5 minutes.

2. Cut the aubergine in half lengthways, add a little salt and lemon juice and return this to the microwave for about 2 minutes until the aubergine is soft and cooked.

3. Gently scoop out the pulp and seeds into a bowl. Mix this with the turmeric, spring onions, black pepper and chilli powder (if using). Adjust the seasoning and serve either in

a bowl or put the pulp back into the aubergine shell and cover with the 'lid'. Garnish with sprigs of fresh coriander.

Nutrition Nuggets: The aubergine skin will give you fibre and nutrients, so whether you serve the pulp within the aubergine shell or not, do enjoy the skin anyway.

Spicy Baked Beans

I GiP per serving

This dish has quite a kick, so reduce the amount of spices if you prefer a milder recipe.

Serves I

220 g can Tesco Healthy Living baked beans
¼–½ tsp red chilli powder
½ tsp curry powder
I tbsp freshly chopped coriander leaves and stems
¼ tsp ground garam masala
½ tsp cumin seeds, lightly crushed in a pestle and mortar
Black pepper
Dash of Worcester sauce

1. Mix all the ingredients together, add the seasoning to taste and serve hot or cold.

Coriander Chutney

0 GiPs per serving

This chutney can last for a few days in a jar in the fridge, so the recipe makes enough for about 3 servings. A hand blender works wonders for this dish – ready in seconds.

Serves 3

100 g fresh coriander leaves and stems, finely chopped
For the dressing:
2 tbsp lemon juice, or to taste
½ tsp coarse-grain mustard
Coarse black pepper
Generous pinch of red chilli powder
2 tsp soy sauce

1. Mix all the dressing ingredients together in a jar.
2. Add to the chopped coriander and mix well. Taste and add more lemon juice, water or soy sauce if you like it thinner. Store in the refrigerator in a screw-topped jar till needed.

Aromatic Basmati Rice

2.5 GiPs per serving

Boiled rice is a classic accompaniment to many Indian, Chinese and Mexican dishes. However, there's nothing quite like the aroma of whole Indian spices to give basmati rice its special authentic touch.

Serves 2

90 g basmati rice
4 whole black peppercorns
3 cloves
1 cinnamon stick, broken
½ tsp cumin seeds
¼ tsp salt

1. Rinse the rice in warm water and add to a pan containing plenty of boiling water.
2. Add all the other ingredients and cook uncovered over a low heat for about 12–15 minutes, or according to the instructions on the packet. Drain the water and fluff up the rice with a fork.

Nutrition Nuggets: Basmati rice is more compact in structure than other types of rice. This, coupled with its higher amounts of a particular type of slowly digested starch, means it causes a slower blood sugar rise than many other rice varieties.

Wheat-free Tabbouleh

0 GiPs per serving

A great GiP-free recipe to accompany any meal.

Serves 1

2 tbsp chopped flat-leaf parsley
3 tomatoes, diced finely
1 tbsp chopped mint leaves
¼ red onion, finely chopped

For the dressing:

Pinch of ground allspice

Pinch of ground cinnamon

1 tbsp lemon juice

Pinch of salt

Coarse black pepper

1. First make the dressing. Put all the dressing ingredients into a screw-top jar, cover and shake vigorously.
2. Mix together all the other ingredients. Toss in the dressing and serve.

Nutrition Nuggets: There is research to show that cinnamon may help in the management of diabetes, so use it often.

Middle-Eastern Tabbouleh

2 GiPs per serving

A traditional Lebanese salad that combines the interesting texture of bulgur wheat with aromatic herbs and spices.

Serves 1

50 g bulgur wheat, pre-soaked in hot water for 30 minutes, drained

50 g flat-leaf parsley, chopped roughly

15 g mint leaves (chopped), or 1 tbsp dried mint

2 tomatoes, finely diced

½ onion, finely chopped

For the dressing:

Juice of 1 lemon

Pinch of salt
Freshly ground black pepper
Pinch of ground allspice
Pinch of ground cinnamon

1. Stir all the dressing ingredients together.
2. Mix the cooked wheat with the parsley, mint, tomatoes, onions and dressing. Serve chilled.

Nutrition Nuggets: If you're not keen on bulgur wheat, opt for Wheat-free Tabbouleh (see recipe, page 224), but remember it's the low-GI carbs like bulgur wheat that give you the health benefits.

Veg Box

0 GiPs per serving

Throw together any combination of the following: courgette sticks, cucumber sticks, baby gherkins, radishes, cherry tomatoes, celery, baby sweetcorn, sugar snap peas, pickled onions, peppers.

Olive and Cucumber Snack Box

0.5 GiPs per serving

Throw together 10 black or green olives, cucumber sticks, and any combination of the following: celery sticks, radishes, pickled onions, gherkins, water chestnuts.

Chilli and Lime Rocket Leaves

0 GiPs per serving

Mix together your favourite combination of free salad veggies and rocket leaves. Make a dressing using fresh lime juice, paprika, dried herbs and chilli sauce. Drench and devour.

MEAT AND POULTRY

Chilli Chicken on Granary

2.5 GiPs per serving

This is a great recipe when you have leftover cooked chicken in the fridge. It's also a great shortcut to use some supermarket cooked chicken breast. Otherwise, simply cook the chicken breast in a little stock.

Serves I

50 g (about ½ breast) cooked chicken breast, shredded into tiny
   pieces
I tbsp skimmed milk
I tbsp soy sauce
Good pinch of red chilli powder
I tsp curry powder
2 spring onions, chopped
Olive oil spray
I thin slice granary bread

1. Preheat the oven to 200°C. Line an oven tray with foil.
2. Mix the chicken breast with all the other ingredients except the oil and bread.
3. Spray one side of the bread with 5 sprays of oil and place this, oiled side down, on the tray. Pile the chicken mixture onto the bread and bake for 5–10 minutes. Serve hot.

Nutrition Nuggets: If you experiment with flavoursome ingredients such as herbs and spices, you can reduce the need for salt or fat.

Chicken Fajitas

4 GiPs per serving

This dish is one of the Govindji family favourites. We often make it when we have some leftover chicken in the fridge.

Serves 1

Olive oil spray
1 small onion, sliced
¼ green pepper, finely sliced
¼ red pepper, finely sliced
1 tsp crushed ginger
1 tsp crushed garlic
50 g (about ½ breast) cooked chicken, cut into strips
2 tomatoes, chopped
1 green chilli, chopped (deseeded if you want to reduce the heat)
50 ml passata (sieved tomatoes)
1 tortilla wrap
Handful of shredded lettuce leaves
5-cm piece cucumber, cut into strips

1. Heat a non-stick pan and add 10 sprays of oil. Stir in the onion, peppers, ginger and garlic and stir-fry for a few minutes till softened.
2. Add the chicken, tomatoes, chilli, passata and 50 ml of hot water.
3. Heat through, and add seasoning to taste.
4. Warm the tortilla wrap, and pile on the chicken mixture with shredded lettuce and cucumber. Fold into the wrap.

Nutrition Nuggets: This low-fat filling can be served on its own (only 1 GiP) with salad, or accompanied with low-GI couscous or bulgur wheat instead of the wrap. There are several recipes for couscous and bulgur wheat in this chapter.

Citrus Roast Chicken Parcels

3 GiPs per serving

Lemon pepper is delicious in this recipe. It's available in supermarkets, but if you doubt you'll use it again, just use regular coarse black pepper and a dash of lemon juice.

Serves 1

1 large chicken breast, skinned
1 tsp crushed garlic
½ tsp herbes de Provence
A little salt
½ tsp lemon pepper
Olive oil spray
1 small orange, sliced
Good pinch of paprika powder

1. Preheat the oven to 200°C. Cut a square of foil large enough to encase the chicken breast.
2. Place the chicken breast in the foil, and flavour with the garlic, herbs and seasoning. Add 10 sprays of oil on top, and then place the orange slices on the chicken breast.
3. Cover loosely with foil and bake for about 15 minutes.
4. Uncover the chicken, sprinkle on the paprika and baste

the chicken with the juices. Return to the oven to brown for about 5 minutes. Serve hot with the juices drizzled over the top.

Nutrition Nuggets: Skinless chicken breast has one of the lowest levels of fat of any meat around. Try it with sweet potatoes or Garlic Spaghetti with Courgette Ribbons (see recipe, page 258).

Juicy Drumsticks with Roasted Shallots

2 GiPs per serving

I suggest you buy drumsticks with the skin on and remove the skin yourself. You will find it quite difficult to get the final bits of skin from the base of the bone and it's fine to leave a little bit of that skin on to add flavour to this dish. This way, you will need no additional oil – you're not actually eating the skin yet you get lots of flavour. Although shallots have a slightly sweeter taste, you can use half an onion instead.

Serves 2

4 chicken drumsticks, skinned as above
1 heaped tsp coarse-grain mustard
3 tbsp Worcester sauce
1 tsp crushed garlic
1 tsp crushed ginger
1 bay leaf (optional)
Good pinch of dried herbs, e.g. oregano or basil

Salt and pepper
6 shallots, peeled and diced
½ tsp paprika powder

1. Preheat the oven to 220°C. Make a dressing with the mustard, Worcester sauce, garlic, ginger, bay leaf (if using), herbs and seasoning.
2. Place the diced onion into an ovenproof dish and lay the drumsticks on top.
3. Coat the drumsticks with the dressing and sprinkle with paprika.
4. Cover tightly with foil and cook for about 15–20 minutes. Uncover, baste and return to the oven to brown for about 5 minutes or until fully cooked and the juices run clear.

Nutrition Nuggets: Poultry skin is high in saturated fat so it's best to use skinned cuts as in this recipe. Serve with plenty of vegetables and a low-GI carb.

Pan-fried Turkey Breasts with Cajun Spice and Tarragon

3.5 GiPs per serving

The Cajun seasoning gives this dish a wonderful charred appearance. No need to add salt as the seasoning is quite salty.

Serves 1

½ tsp Cajun spice
½ tsp dried mixed herbs
1 tbsp freshly chopped tarragon

½ tsp paprika seasoning
Coarse black pepper
1 skinless turkey breast, weighing around 170 g
1 tsp olive or rapeseed oil

1. Mix together the Cajun spice, herbs, tarragon, paprika and pepper. Sprinkle this mixture over both sides of the turkey.
2. Heat a non-stick frying pan and add the oil. Pan-fry the flavoured turkey breast over a medium heat for about 5–8 minutes, turn the breast over and cook the other side for about 5 minutes, till the turkey is fully cooked.

Nutrition Nuggets: Turkey breast, as with other poultry, is very low in fat. The skin, however, is high in saturated fat, so it's best to get into the habit of removing the skin before cooking. Serve with low-GiP accompaniments such as pasta or bulgur wheat and piles of colourful vegetables.

Turkey (or Chicken) and Almond Koftas with Warm Plum Chutney

2.5 GiPs per serving

This exotic-sounding dish couldn't be easier. If you have a food processor, it takes about a minute to blitz all the ingredients together. All you need to do then is to make the koftas into sausage shapes. If you don't have a food processor, use minced turkey breast, chopped almonds, crushed garlic and diced onions and just mix the ingredients together.

Makes 20 koftas, 4 servings

For the koftas:

450 g turkey (or chicken) breast pieces

25 g almonds

3 garlic cloves, peeled

30 g parsley or coriander leaves with stems

1 slice granary bread, broken into large pieces

1 egg

1 small onion, cut into quarters

Salt and pepper

Pinch of dried herbs of your choice

To sprinkle on shaped koftas:

Paprika or red chilli powder

For the plum chutney:

3 plums, stoned and diced into chunks

150 ml hot water

Good pinch of red chilli powder

Good pinch of salt

1 cinnamon stick or pinch of ground cinnamon

Juice of 1 medium orange

1 tbsp lemon juice

To serve:

Fresh salad leaves

1. Preheat the grill and line a grill pan with foil.
2. Put all the kofta ingredients into a food processor and blitz for only about a minute to mix all the ingredients together. Make sure you don't over-process as the final mixture should still have small chunks of nuts and turkey.
3. Shape the flavoured turkey mixture into 20 sausage shapes, about 8 cm in length. Place them in one layer on the lined grill pan.

4. Sprinkle with paprika or red chilli powder and grill for 5–10 minutes until browned and cooked, turning once.

5. Meanwhile, prepare the plum chutney by placing all the ingredients into a non-stick pan. Cook the chutney ingredients over a medium heat until softened but still chunky, about 10 minutes.

6. Serve the koftas on a bed of mixed salad leaves with the chutney.

Nutrition Nuggets: Turkey and chicken are both low-fat meats, and this recipe requires no additional cooking oil. Both the almonds and the plums are nutritious low-GI ingredients.

Creamy Tagliatelli with Ham (or Chilli Beans) and Field Mushrooms

4 GiPs per serving

When you make pasta without added oil, it can sometimes taste quite dry. A good trick is to keep some of the hot water in the pan when you are draining the pasta. Then cover with a lid and this will allow the pasta to stay moist. Field mushrooms add a distinctive flavour to this dish, but you can choose regular mushrooms if you prefer. For a vegetarian option, substitute the ham with chilli beans.

Serves I

50 g egg *tagliatelli*
Olive oil spray
½ *onion, finely sliced*
I *tsp crushed garlic*

100 g French beans, boiled

100 g field mushrooms, sliced

15 g fresh basil leaves, torn

Salt and pepper

50 g cooked ham, chopped, or ¼ can chilli beans

100 ml Greek sheep's yoghurt or low-fat Greek-style yoghurt

1. Cook the pasta in lightly salted boiling water until *al dente* (firm to the bite). Drain (not quite fully), cover and keep warm.

2. Heat a non-stick pan over a medium heat and add 10 sprays of oil. Stir-fry the onion and garlic for a couple of minutes to soften, adding a couple of tablespoons of hot water if they begin to stick to the bottom.

3. Stir in the French beans and mushrooms and cook for a few minutes. Flavour with the basil leaves and seasoning.

4. Mix in the drained pasta and ham (or chilli beans). Heat through, stir in the Greek yoghurt, add seasoning to taste and serve. Do not overheat.

Nutrition Nuggets: The more *al dente* you can keep cooked pasta, the lower its GI is likely to be. If you prefer a richer sauce, choose 50 ml half-fat crème fraîche and add 1 GiP per serving.

Beefier Burgers

3 GiPs per serving

Homemade burgers are full of texture and goodness. They are likely to contain far more beef than any fast-food burger you could find, and you know exactly what's in them! They are grilled but you could dry-fry them in a griddle pan if you prefer. There is plenty of juice to keep them moist.

Serves 1

½ slice granary bread
150 g lean minced beef
½ onion, grated
½ egg, beaten
½ tsp curry powder
Good pinch of red chilli powder, optional
¼ tsp mustard
Pinch of salt

1. Preheat the grill to medium. Run some cold water over the bread and squeeze out the excess. Mix the soaked bread with all the other ingredients, either in a food processor or by hand, and shape into one large or two small burgers.
2. Place directly onto the rack of the grill-pan to allow the fat to drain away during cooking. Grill each side for 5–7 minutes or until cooked through.

Nutrition Nuggets: Regular hamburger buns cause a rapid rise in blood sugar and therefore have a high-GI value. Instead, serve these burgers with a lower-GI carb, such as Spicy Baked Beans (see recipe, page 222), Warburtons All In One Rolls, Simple Bulgur Wheat (see recipe, page 215) and masses of salad vegetables. Remember to add the GiPs from your accompaniments.

Chilli Con Carne

4.5 GiPs per serving

Serves I

Spray oil

I small onion, finely chopped

Good pinch of cumin seeds

I tsp crushed garlic

I green chilli, deseeded and chopped

150 ml canned chopped tomatoes

125 g lean minced beef

½ can kidney beans, drained

15 g flat leaf parsley, roughly chopped

Salt and pepper, to taste

1. Heat a non-stick pan and add 10 sprays of oil. Gently sauté the chopped onion in the oil, adding a couple of tablespoons of hot water if they begin to stick to the bottom.

2. Add the cumin seeds, garlic, chilli and chopped tomatoes. Stir and allow to cook for a few minutes.

3. Add the minced beef with some more hot water (or tomato juice from the canned tomatoes) if needed. Stir well, cover and cook for about 10–15 minutes.

4. Stir in the kidney beans and continue cooking for a few minutes until the beef is fully cooked.

5. Add the flat leaf parsley, season to taste and serve.

Nutrition Nuggets: It may surprise you to know that beans are actually a carbohydrate. Since they are a low-GI carb, you may choose to simply have this dish with a salad. Alternatively, serve with bulgur wheat (see recipes in this chapter), steamed Basmati or brown rice (see tables for GiP value).

Beef Chow Mein

4 GiPs per serving

Have a Chinese take-away at home with this flavoursome noodle dish packed with low-GI ingredients.

Serves 4

Spray oil
400 g beef steak, cut into thin strips
1 onion, thinly sliced
1 heaped tsp crushed ginger
1 tsp crushed garlic
3–4 tbsp soy sauce
1 tsp five-spice powder
½–1 tsp dried basil
170 g mangetout
1 can baby corn, drained and sliced or cut in half lengthways
150 g mushrooms, sliced
1 red pepper, thinly sliced
200 g medium egg noodles
200 g beansprouts
Salt and pepper
To serve:
2 spring onions, green stems only, sliced diagonally
1 tbsp plum sauce or sweet chilli sauce

1. Heat a non-stick wok and spray with 10 sprays of oil. Stir-fry the beef for two minutes before adding the onion, ginger and garlic. Fry for a further 5 minutes.
2. Add all the flavourings and vegetables and stir-fry for about 3 minutes until the beef is cooked.
3. Meanwhile, cook the noodles according to the instructions on the packet.
4. Stir the beansprouts into the wok, heat through and adjust soy sauce and seasoning.
5. Serve the stir-fried beef either on a bed of noodles or mix the noodles together with the beef in the wok and adjust seasoning if necessary.
6. Serve garnished with sliced spring onion and drizzled with plum sauce or sweet chilli sauce.

Nutrition Nuggets: You get around two of your five-a-day vegetable recommendations from just one serving of this dish. Choose lean beef to keep the saturated fat down.

Minty Lamb Chops on Roasted Apple Rings

2 GiPs per serving

It takes less than a minute to dress these chops and under 15 minutes to cook in a hot oven. If you prefer, you can grill on both sides until the juices run clear.

Serves 1

1 Granny Smith apple, cored and sliced into rings

2 lean lamb chops

Ground black pepper

1½ tsp mint sauce

½ tsp dried oregano

½ tsp vegetable bouillon powder

1. Preheat the oven to 220°C. Line an oven tray with foil, or use a non-stick oven tray and place the apple rings in a single layer on the tray. Season the chops with ground black pepper and lay these on top of the apple rings.

2. Mix together the mint sauce, oregano and vegetable bouillon powder and spread this paste over the top of the chops.

3. Bake for 12–15 minutes until fully cooked and the juices run clear.

Nutrition Nuggets: This is a speedy way of getting iron, zinc and vitamin B12 from these lean lamb chops, as well as a portion of your five-a-day recommended fruit and vegetables. You don't need to add salt as the boullion powder is quite salty.

FISH DISHES

Stuffed Mackerel

2.5 GiPs per serving

You can use this recipe for plain baked mackerel, too. The GiPs will be the same and you will still get the valuable omega-3 fats from the fish. Ask your fishmonger or supermarket to clean the inside of the fish and remove the scales.

Serves 2

2 whole mackerel
1–2 cloves fresh garlic, sliced, as desired
1 small tomato, chopped finely
4 spring onions, sliced
½ green pepper, chopped finely
1 tbsp lemon juice
4 tbsp freshly chopped dill
A little salt and pepper

1. Heat the oven to 180°C and line an oven tray with foil or use a non-stick roasting tin. Make diagonal slits in the mackerel and slot the garlic slices into the slits.
2. Lay the mackerel on the foil or tin. Mix together the tomato, onions, green pepper, lemon juice and dill and use this mixture to stuff the fish, placing any remaining stuffing next to the fish.
3. Season lightly, cover with foil and bake for about 10–15 minutes till cooked. Serve with the baked stuffing and juices.

Nutrition Nuggets: The acidic lemon juice and vegetables help to keep the GI of any accompanying carbs low. You don't need to add any oil to this dish as you get plenty of natural fish oils from the mackerel.

Potato, Apple and Tuna Salad

4.5 GiPs per serving

A substantial portion for hungry days.

Serves 1

4 new potatoes, scrubbed
½ can tuna in brine, drained
1 apple, chopped
½ stick celery, sliced (optional)
75 ml Greek sheep's yoghurt
½ tsp mint sauce
Handful of snipped chives
Handful of freshly chopped dill
Cracked black pepper

1. Boil the new potatoes in lightly salted boiling water in a covered saucepan till just cooked.
2. Chop the potatoes into bite-size pieces.
3. Mix with all the other ingredients, season to taste as necessary. Leave to cool and chill in the refrigerator till needed.

Nutrition Nuggets: Potatoes tend to have a medium- to high-GI value. New potatoes in their skins offer one of the lowest-GI values for potatoes. It may surprise you to know that cooled cooked potatoes promote a lower blood-glucose response than hot ones. So, potato salad as in this recipe, especially when mixed with the other low-GI ingredients, makes an excellent lower-GI meal.

Tandoori Prawns

1.5 GiPs per serving

A great low-fat filling for wraps, pitta bread or with a simple crisp green salad. If you have time, leave the prawns in the tandoori marinade for about 20 minutes before cooking.

Serves 1

125 g cooked prawns
½ tsp tandoori powder or paste
1 tsp tomato purée
75 ml low-fat natural yoghurt
Olive oil spray
½–1 tsp cumin seeds
1 tbsp chopped coriander leaves
Few leaves Romaine lettuce, shredded
5-cm piece cucumber, cut into sticks

1. Mix together the prawns, tandoori flavouring, tomato purée and low-fat natural yoghurt.
2. Heat a heavy-based non-stick frying pan to medium and add 10 sprays of oil. Fry the cumin seeds for a few seconds, being careful not to let them burn.

3. Quickly stir in the marinated prawns and cook over a moderate heat till the liquid is reduced and begins to thicken.
4. Stir in the coriander leaves and serve the tandoori prawns, hot or cold, on a bed of lettuce and cucumber.

Nutrition Nuggets: Although prawns do contain cholesterol, it is actually the saturated fat in your diet that has a significant influence on your blood cholesterol levels, rather than the cholesterol itself. Although wholemeal pitta bread will not have a significantly different GI value from white, it does offer you more fibre.

Sesame Prawn Toasts

2.5 GiPs per serving

Serves 1

60 g cooked prawns
½ egg white
1–2 tsp Chinese five-spice powder, as desired
Black pepper
Few drops of sesame oil
Olive oil spray
1 slice Warburtons All In One or granary bread
1 tsp sesame seeds
To serve:
Crisp salad leaves drizzled with lemon juice
Lemon wedges

1. Preheat the oven to 190°C. Line an oven tray with foil or use a non-stick tray.
2. Mash the prawns and blend with the egg white, either by hand or using an electric blender.
3. Season with the five-spice powder, pepper and sesame oil.
4. Spray one side of the bread with 5 sprays of oil. Lay the bread, oiled side down, onto the tray and spread the prawn mixture on top, pressing down lightly.
5. Top with sesame seeds and bake in the oven for about 12–15 minutes or till crisp. Cut into quarters and serve with crisp salad leaves and fresh lemon wedges.

Nutrition Nuggets: Prawn toast that you might order in a Chinese restaurant is likely to be deep-fried and so high in fat. This healthier method simply uses a hot oven to crisp up the toast and cook the prawns.

Tuna (or Egg) Niçoise

2 GiPs per serving

The ingredients in this list are appropriate for a tuna niçoise. If you prefer a vegetarian version of this recipe, simply transform this into an egg 'niçoise' by substituting the tuna with one extra boiled egg.

Serves 1

Generous handful of mixed salad leaves
6–8 cherry tomatoes or 3 or 4 firm tomatoes, cut into wedges
125 g cooked French beans

Small can tuna in brine, drained

1 boiled egg, cut into wedges

10 black or green olives

Small handful of fresh basil leaves, torn

2 tbsp fat-free dressing (e.g. fat-free Thousand Island dressing)

Ground black pepper

1. Lay the salad leaves on a plate and arrange the tomatoes, beans, tuna and/or egg, olives and basil leaves on top.
2. Drizzle with the dressing and flavour with ground black pepper.

Nutrition Nuggets: You can make this into a fantastic main meal by mixing in, or serving on a bed of, Simple Bulgur Wheat (see recipe, page 215), a delicious low-GI carb.

Thai-style Trout with Basil and Ginger

1.5 GiPs per serving

You can use any fish for this recipe, but it works particularly well with trout or salmon. You can use any oven-proof dish to cook this, but to ensure it doesn't stick, line with foil or use a non-stick dish or tray.

Serves 1

1 fillet fresh trout

½ tsp crushed ginger

2 tbsp Thai fish sauce

Handful of basil leaves, finely chopped
1 green chilli, deseeded and chopped
Olive oil spray
1 lime, cut into wedges

1. Preheat the oven to 200°C and line an oven tray with foil. Lay the trout on the foil. Flavour the trout with the ginger, fish sauce, basil leaves and chilli.
2. Add 5 sprays of oil and bake in the oven for about 10–12 minutes. Serve immediately, garnished with fresh lime.

Nutrition Nuggets: Oily fish such as trout are packed with nutritious omega-3 fats. These essential fats help to reduce the risk of heart disease.

Lemony Cod Strips with Spicy Bulgur Wheat

3 GiPs per serving

A great low-GI dish to have when entertaining. Simply increase the ingredients accordingly if cooking for a family. Accompany with some lightly steamed broccoli or other GiP-free vegetables of your choice. If you want to make it really special, garnish with 6 sliced toasted almonds per fillet (the finished dish will provide 4.5 GiPs per serving). The fish is cooking while you put the bulgur wheat on the boil, so the whole meal takes about 20–25 minutes.

Serves 1

Olive oil spray

Salt and pepper

1 cod fillet, fresh or frozen (weighing about 175 g)

Few sprigs of lemon thyme

¼ tsp herbes de Provence

2 tsp lemon juice

For the Spicy Bulgur Wheat:

50 g bulgur wheat

*200 ml vegetable stock (made with ½ stock cube and 200 ml
    boiling water)*

Good pinch of ground turmeric

3 whole black peppercorns

1 cinnamon stick, broken

Good pinch of garam masala

¼–½ tsp hot red chilli powder, to taste

½ tsp ground coriander

Handful of fresh mint or coriander leaves, chopped (optional)

½ fresh lime, cut into wedges

1. Heat the grill and line a grill pan with foil. Add 5 sprays of
    oil, season and place the cod fillets directly onto the
    flavoured oil.
2. Remove the thyme leaves from the stalks and scatter
    these over the cod. Sprinkle the dried herbs on top and
    add seasoning.
3. Drizzle with lemon juice, add 5 more sprays of oil and grill
    under a moderate heat for 12–15 minutes, turning once
    during cooking.
4. Meanwhile, put the bulgur wheat and vegetable stock into
    a non-stick pan and bring back to the boil.

5. Stir in the turmeric, peppercorns, cinnamon stick, garam masala, chilli powder and ground coriander. Simmer for 12–15 minutes till all the water is absorbed and the wheat is cooked.

6. Stir the fresh herbs (if using) into the cooked bulgur, add seasoning to taste and lay on a warmed plate.

7. Cut the cod into strips and lay these on top of the wheat. Garnish with fresh lime wedges.

Nutrition Nuggets: Barley has the lowest GI of any grain, followed closely by bulgur wheat. Brown rice and basmati rice are next, with a slightly higher GI. So, when a recipe calls for rice, either choose these low-GI rice examples or, better still, opt for bulgur wheat. Add a generous serving of green vegetables or a side salad.

Tuna Pasta Salad

4 GiPs per serving

A lunchtime favourite, and one that you would probably buy from a store. Try this for a cheaper and probably even healthier option. Simple ingredients that you put together in about 10–15 minutes.

Serves 1

50 g pasta shells (or other shaped pasta of your choice)
1 can tuna in brine, drained
¼ red onion, chopped (optional)
1 tbsp canned sweetcorn

1 stick celery, sliced (optional)
5-cm stick cucumber, diced
Handful of basil leaves, shredded
Good pinch of mixed dried herbs
2 tbsp fat-free Thousand Island dressing
Generous pinch of black or cayenne pepper

1. Cook the pasta shells in lightly salted boiling water until *al dente* (firm to the bite). Drain and leave aside to cool.
2. Mix the pasta with the tuna, onion (if using), sweetcorn, celery (if using), cucumber, herbs and dressing. Stir well, season to taste and serve chilled.

Nutrition Nuggets: You can add any GiP-free vegetables to bulk up this dish if you like. Check out the tables (page 293) for suggestions.

VEGETABLE MAINS

Baked Flat Mushrooms with Melted Camembert

3 GiPs per serving

Go to a fancy restaurant and you may be served this dish drenched in olive oil and topped with a tower of goat's cheese. Both of these ingredients are rich in fat, and the goat's cheese will add the less-healthy saturated fat – not such a good idea when you're watching your waistline. Instead, opt for this lower-calorie but equally scrumptious dish.

Impress your mates. Simply double up the ingredients if you are making this for two people.

Serves 1

2 large flat mushrooms, washed
Olive oil spray
1 tsp crushed garlic
4 tsp fresh thyme leaves
2 tomatoes, thickly sliced
Salt and black pepper
25 g Camembert cheese, sliced finely
To serve:
Handful of rocket leaves
Handful of Romaine lettuce, torn
Drizzle of balsamic vinegar

1. Preheat the oven to 200°C. Line an ovenproof tray with foil. Remove the stalks from the mushrooms so that you have more space for the filling.

2. Spray the base of each mushroom with 5 sprays of oil. Lay the mushrooms, rounded side down, on the foil and stuff the garlic (if using) and thyme leaves into the mushrooms. Place the stalks next to the mushrooms on the foil.

3. Lay the sliced tomatoes on top of the mushrooms (you will probably have some side bits left – use these to nibble on!) Season with salt and pepper.

4. Bake in the oven for 10 minutes.

5. Remove the mushrooms from the oven; lay the slices of Camembert on top, cutting the cheese to fit, as necessary.

6. Return to the oven for another 5 minutes till the cheese has melted. Serve immediately on the salad leaves flavoured with balsamic vinegar.

Nutrition Nuggets: The acid from the balsamic vinegar and the salad vegetables help to keep the GI low. The Camembert cheese provides fewer calories than Brie, Cheddar or even Edam.

Quorn and Chick Pea Curry

2 GiPs per serving

A great vegetarian curry that offers calorie savings, good sources of protein and lots of fibre. You can serve this with Basmati rice, chapatti, tortilla wrap or pitta bread. Alternatively, accompany the dish with piles of salad or GiP-free vegetables.

East meets West recipe. Takes about 15 minutes.

Serves 1

Olive oil spray
1 small onion, finely chopped
1 heaped tsp cumin seeds
½ tsp crushed ginger
2 cloves garlic, sliced
1 green chilli, deseeded and chopped
1 cinnamon stick, optional
½ can chopped tomatoes or 250 ml passata (sieved tomatoes)
12 pieces of fresh or defrosted Quorn (weighing around 65 g)
60 g/¼ can chick peas, drained
Good pinch of turmeric
Good pinch of ground garam masala
Pinch of salt
100 ml hot water
15 g coriander leaves and stems, roughly chopped

1. Heat a heavy-based non-stick frying pan and then add 10 sprays of oil. Reduce the heat to medium and stir in the onion and cumin seeds, and allow to fry for 1 minute.
2. Add the ginger, garlic, chilli and cinnamon stick (if using), and stir well to allow the aroma to develop.
3. Add the tomatoes, Quorn, chick peas, turmeric, garam masala and salt. Stir for a few minutes till lightly blended.
4. Pour in the water, lower the heat, cover and simmer for about 10 minutes.
5. Stir in the chopped coriander leaves, add seasoning to taste and serve hot.

Nutrition Nuggets: Chick peas provide healthy soluble fibre, which can help lower blood cholesterol. Since the chick peas are kept whole (as opposed to mashed up in a dish like hummus), you are able to keep the GI lower.

Savoury French Toast

5 GiPs per serving

A delicious breakfast, which only takes about 5 minutes. One serving will make four triangles of toast, so you may choose to have three of these at breakfast and save one for your mid-morning snack. Also makes a nice supper dish – just add a salad.

Serves 1

2 heaped tbsp chopped fresh coriander leaves
Good pinch of mustard or ½ tsp coarse-grain mustard
Pinch of salt
Coarse black pepper
2 slices granary bread, cut into four halves
2 eggs, beaten
Olive oil spray
Worcester sauce, as desired

1. Mix the coriander leaves, mustard, salt and pepper with the eggs. Soak both sides of the bread in this egg mixture.
2. Heat a non-stick frying pan or wok. Add 5 to 10 sprays of oil and gently fry the soaked bread over a medium heat, for 1–2 minutes per side.

3. Drain on kitchen paper and drizzle with Worcester sauce. Serve hot or cold.

Nutrition Nuggets: Regular French toast uses white bread and oil for frying. This clever recipe lowers the GI by using granary bread and lowers the fat by using spray oil. Just as delicious, but miles better for you!

Greek Salad

3 GiPs per serving

Serves 1

10 olives, halved
10 cherry tomatoes
2 handfuls of mixed salad leaves (100–150 g)
2 tbsp fat-free dressing
½ red onion, sliced (optional)
Good pinch of mixed herbs
25 g feta cheese, cut into small chunks

1. Mix together all the ingredients except the feta cheese.
2. Lay the feta on top of the salad.

Nutrition Nuggets: Substituting a standard oily dressing with a fat-free version helps to keep the calories low, so you focus on taste, not your waist!

Fettuccine with Creamy Spinach Sauce and Marinated Tomatoes

3.5 GiPs per serving

Serves 1

2 tomatoes, cut into wedges
2 tbsp lemon juice
Coarse black pepper
A little salt
50 g egg fettuccine
½ tsp crushed garlic
125 g baby spinach leaves
Olive oil spray
½ onion, finely chopped
Good pinch of dried oregano
Good pinch of dried rosemary
50 ml half-fat crème fraîche

1. Marinate the tomatoes in the lemon juice, black pepper
    and salt, while you are preparing the rest of the dish.
2. Boil the pasta in lightly salted boiling water until *al dente*
    (firm to the bite), according to the packet instructions.
    Drain, but leave around a tablespoon of water in the
    pot with the pasta. Stir in the crushed garlic, cover and
    keep warm.
3. Wilt the spinach leaves by immersing them in around
    1 cm of boiling water, cover with a tight-fitting lid and
    steam over a high heat for a maximum of 2–3 minutes.
4. Heat a non-stick pan, and add 10 sprays of oil. Lightly
    sauté the onion and dried herbs.

5. Stir in the drained spinach and when warm, add the crème fraîche. Do not boil. Season to taste.

6. Place a bed of garlic fettuccine on a plate, and lay the creamy spinach on top. Lastly, place the marinated tomatoes on the spinach, and drizzle any left-over marinade over the pasta. Serve immediately.

Nutrition Nuggets: Different colours of vegetables will provide a wider range of nutrients – the spinach and tomatoes in this dish offer vibrant colours as well as valuable beta-carotene, folic acid and vitamin C.

Garlic Spaghetti with Courgette Ribbons

3 GiPs per serving

Serves 1

50 g (around 60 strands) raw spaghetti
2 courgettes, topped and tailed
1 tsp olive oil
2 tsp crushed garlic
½ onion, finely chopped
2 tbsp freshly chopped parsley
A little salt
Freshly ground black pepper

1. Cook the spaghetti in lightly salted boiling water until *al dente* (firm to the bite), according to the packet instructions. Drain and keep warm.

2. Meanwhile, cut the courgettes into ribbons using a

Y-shaped vegetable peeler, and steam in a covered pan for a few minutes using a minimum of boiling water.

3. Heat the olive oil in a non-stick pan. Stir in the garlic and onions and sauté till soft. Add a tablespoon or two of hot water if the onions begin to stick to the bottom of the pan.

4. Add the cooked spaghetti, courgettes and parsley. Heat through, season and serve.

Nutrition Nuggets: Pasta is one of the best low-GI carbs. It's great for athletes who want to load up with carbohydrate before an event, and it's a fantastic everyday food that fills you up and is also low in calories. Choose wholemeal varieties for added fibre.

Green Lentil Dahl/Main Meal Dahl and Peanut Soup

I GiP per serving/4 GiPs per serving

This clever version of a traditional Indian dish uses canned lentils from the Cheat's Whole Lentil and Coriander Soup recipe to give you authenticity in minutes. Simply follow the instructions for the soup (see recipe, page 207) and then use this soup to create your aromatic dahl dish. Or make enough soup for two servings, and enjoy the soup at one sitting and spice the rest up into a dahl for another time.

For a Main Meal Dahl and Peanut Soup (4 GiPs),
simply throw in 25 g of chopped peanuts at
Step 2 and add more water if desired.

Serves 1

Olive oil spray
½ tsp black mustard seeds
½ tsp cumin seeds
½ tsp chopped ginger
1 portion of Cheat's Whole Lentil and Coriander Soup (page 207)
1 green chilli, sliced (remove seeds for less heat)
¼ tsp ground turmeric
¼ tsp ground garam masala
2 spring onions, green stems only, sliced
2 tbsp chopped coriander leaves and stems
(For the Dahl and Peanut Soup: 25 g peanuts, chopped)

1. Heat a non-stick pan and add 10 sprays of oil. Lower the heat to a minimum and throw in the mustard and cumin seeds. Allow to pop for just a few seconds before adding the ginger and the prepared soup.
2. Stir in the chilli, turmeric and garam masala and cook through for a few minutes.
3. Add the spring onions and coriander leaves and serve.

Nutrition Nuggets: Dahls are a great way to sneak well-flavoured lentils into your menu. Cooking them from dry has a slightly lower GI, but canned lentils are also fantastic.

Creamy Tagliatelli with Chilli Beans and Field Mushrooms

4 GiPs per serving

See page 235.

10-minute Mushroom Stroganoff

I GiP per serving

This mouthwatering vegetarian recipe can be conjured up in minutes and tastes wonderfully creamy.

Serves I

Olive oil spray
¼ onion, finely diced
I tsp crushed garlic
125 g button mushrooms, washed
3 tbsp chopped flat-leaf parsley
150 ml low-fat yoghurt or Greek sheep's yoghurt

1. Heat a non-stick frying pan or wok over a moderate heat and add 10 sprays of oil. Stir fry the onion and garlic, adding 2–3 tbsp of hot water if the mixture begins to stick to the bottom.
2. Add the mushrooms and flat-leaf parsley and cook for 3–4 minutes. Meanwhile, beat the yoghurt with a teaspoon until creamy.
3. Season well, lower the heat and stir in the yoghurt. Remove from the heat to prevent the yoghurt from curdling and serve.

Nutrition Nuggets: Best served with a low-GI carb such as brown rice, Simple Bulgur Wheat (see recipe, page 215) or spicy bulgur wheat (see recipe for Lemony Cod Strips with Spicy Bulgur Wheat, page 249). Add a crispy side salad for balance.

Nutty Couscous with Lime and Parsley

5 GiPs per serving

If you like a bit of crunch, then this recipe is likely to be one of your favourites.

Serves 1

Olive oil spray
60 g couscous
60 ml vegetable stock (made up using ½ stock cube and 60 ml
*   hot water)*
15 g salted peanuts
Juice from ½ fresh lime
Generous handful of parsley, roughly chopped
1 spring onion, green stems only, sliced
Salt and pepper

1. Heat a non-stick saucepan and add 10 sprays of oil. Add the couscous and stir-fry for about 2 minutes.
2. Stir in the stock, cover and remove from the heat. Set aside for 5 minutes to allow the water to be absorbed.
3. Meanwhile, heat a frying pan and dry-roast the peanuts for less than a minute, stirring frequently to prevent burning. Chop the peanuts if you prefer, before or after roasting.
4. When the couscous is cooked, add the peanuts, lime juice, parsley and spring onions. Return to the heat for 3–4 minutes, fluff up with a fork and season to taste. Serve hot or cold.

Nutrition Nuggets: Couscous is a medium-GI food. Use it as an accompaniment to chicken or fish, or even on its own as a vegetarian main meal. Add a side salad or some steamed vegetables for balance.

Vegetable Pasta in Rich Tomato and Basil Sauce

4.5 GiPs per serving

Pasta is one of the most versatile low-GI carbs. It can be served hot or cold, mixed with vegetables or meat, or simply served as a side dish to a main meal. This recipe uses a low-fat homemade tomato sauce, which is better for your waistline than a traditional cheese sauce.

Serves 1

50 g pasta shells
1 tsp olive oil
1 tsp crushed garlic
1 small onion, finely chopped
½ green pepper, finely diced
½ red pepper, finely diced
200 ml passata (sieved tomatoes)
½ tsp dried oregano
1 large courgette, sliced
Generous handful basil leaves, torn into small pieces
2 tomatoes, chopped
Salt and pepper
1 spring onion, green stems only, sliced

1. Boil the pasta in lightly salted boiling water for about 10 minutes or until *al dente* (firm to the bite).
2. Heat a non-stick pan and add 1 tsp of olive oil. Stir-fry the garlic, onion and peppers in the oil for 3–4 minutes.
3. Stir in the sieved tomatoes with the oregano and courgettes and sauté for a few minutes. Add 2–3 tbsp of hot water if the vegetables begin to stick to the bottom.
4. Stir in the basil leaves and add the drained pasta and chopped tomatoes. Cover and cook over a low heat for 3–4 minutes till the flavour has penetrated the pasta.
5. Season to taste, and garnish with chopped spring onions.

Nutrition Nuggets: Tomatoes contain a powerful antioxidant called lycopene. The good news is that, unlike most nutrients, when you process tomatoes you make the lycopene even more concentrated. So this recipe, which uses bought sieved tomatoes as well as fresh crunchy vegetables, is oozing with cancer-fighting antioxidants.

Spinach and Ricotta Cannelloni

4 GiPs per serving

This mouthwatering and tempting meal brings the flavour and colours of the Mediterranean into your own kitchen. It's cheap and easy to make and is a fun way to get the kids cooking in the kitchen. Most recipes in this book can be on the table within 20 minutes. However, because this recipe requires the dried pasta to cook in the oven, you will need to allow about 45 minutes in total.

Serves 1

100 g frozen leaf spinach
Olive oil spray
150 ml tomato-based pasta sauce (preferably reduced-fat)
50 g/4 cannelloni tubes, dried
100 g ricotta cheese
¼ tsp garlic
Good pinch of dried oregano
1 spring onion, sliced
Handful of basil leaves
Salt and freshly ground black pepper

1. Preheat the oven to 220°C. Steam the spinach in around 1 cm of lightly salted boiling water in a covered pan for around 4–5 minutes, or until just cooked.
2. Put 10 sprays of oil in a flat ovenproof dish, wide enough to hold four of the cannelloni tubes in one layer. Spoon about 3 tbsp of the pasta sauce into the dish.
3. Drain the cooked spinach and use around 50 ml of the cooking water to dilute the remaining pasta sauce. This will help to provide adequate moisture to cook the dried pasta.
4. Reserve a few spring onion slices and whole basil leaves for garnish. Mix the ricotta cheese, drained cooked spinach, garlic, oregano, spring onion and torn basil leaves together. Taste and add seasoning.
5. Stuff the cannelloni tubes with the ricotta and spinach filling using a small spoon (a ½ tsp cough mixture measure works really well). If you have any mixture left over, set aside for later.

6. Lay the filled cannelloni onto the pasta sauce in the dish and coat with the remaining pasta sauce. Dollop any leftover mixture on top of this and bake for 20–25 minutes till cooked.
7. Serve hot, scattered with the remaining spring onion and basil.

Nutrition Nuggets: Tomato-based sauces are generally much lower in fat and calories than cheese-based varieties. Compare labels and choose those with less fat per 100 g.

Red Lentil Dahl with Lime and Coriander

I GiP per serving

This easy recipe uses authentic ground spices that you can buy from the supermarket. Dried lentils are a cheap and easy way to have a protein-rich, healthy vegetarian meal. Serve with boiled brown or basmati rice. This dish goes particularly well with Aromatic Basmati Rice (see recipe, page 223) and Speedy Cucumber and Mint Raita (see recipe, page 213). Remember to count the GiPs from the accompaniments. Use a pressure cooker if you're in a rush – follow the manufacturer's instructions for lentils.

Serves I

Olive oil spray
½ onion, finely chopped
½ tsp crushed garlic
½ tsp crushed ginger
100 g canned chopped tomatoes

¼–½ tsp red chilli powder

Pinch of ground garam masala

¼ tsp ground coriander

Pinch of turmeric

50 g dried red lentils

100–150 ml hot water

Salt, to taste

Juice of ½ fresh lime

1 spring onion, green stems only, chopped

1 tbsp roughly chopped coriander leaves and stems

1. Heat a non-stick lidded pan and add 10 sprays of oil. Gently stir-fry the onion, garlic and ginger in the oil, adding a few tablespoons of hot water if the mixture begins to stick to the bottom.

2. Stir in the tomatoes and ground spices. Simmer for 2–3 minutes.

3. Add the lentils and 100 ml hot water. Cover and simmer over a medium heat for about 15 minutes until the dahl is cooked but not mushy. Add a little more hot water if you prefer more sauce.

4. To serve, stir in the salt, lime juice, spring onion and coriander leaves. Taste and add seasoning and chilli as desired.

Nutrition Nuggets: The lentils in this dish are high in soluble fibre. This type of fibre can help lower blood-cholesterol levels. Add this to the lycopene-rich tomatoes and you have a healthy aromatic Indian take-way at home! Keep the lentils cooked but not mushy as this keeps the GI low, and serve with brown or basmati rice.

SWEET THINGS

Spiced Pear with Ginger Fromage Frais

I GiP per serving

Serves I

Olive oil spray

I pear, cored and quartered

Pinch of ground cinnamon

50 ml virtually fat-free fromage frais

Pinch of ginger powder or ¼ tsp finely grated fresh root ginger

Sprig of mint, for garnish

Small amount of icing sugar, for dusting

Orange zest (optional)

1. Heat a non-stick frying pan and add 5 sprays of oil.
2. Soften the pear over a medium heat, adding a little lemon juice if it begins to stick to the bottom. Flavour with a pinch of ground cinnamon.
3. Mix the ginger with the fromage frais and serve with the warm pears. Decorate with a sprig of mint, a dusting of icing sugar and grated orange zest (if using).

Nutrition Nuggets: Virtually fat-free fromage frais contains only about a quarter of the calories of single cream. You can use either a plain or fruity variety for this dish.

Mango Smoothie

2 GiPs per serving

This recipe has been created by Shazia, aged 13, who says '...it's a great way to get two of your five fruits a day and some calcium...and it's way tastier than juice you'd get from a carton.' If you have a smoothie-maker, follow the manufacturer's instructions. Otherwise, just use a blender.

Serves 2

1 small mango, peeled
3 plums peeled and stoned, halved
200 ml semi-skimmed milk
100 ml low-fat yoghurt

1. Chop the mango into large pieces and put it into a blender with all the other ingredients.
2. Blitz in the blender until smooth and creamy. Serve chilled.

Nutrition Nuggets: Smoothies often contain added sugar or honey, but you can usually get enough natural sweetness from the fruit.

Frozen Yoghurt Sticks

1 GiP per serving

I learnt this simple trick while sweltering in the market stalls of Morocco. I noticed freezers stocked with fruit yoghurts that had a stick peeking out over the top. What a great way to cool down! You can use this borrowed trick and enjoy frozen yoghurt ice lollies or, if you prefer, just freeze the yoghurt as it is and have it in the pot as a cold refreshing dessert. It doesn't have quite the same creamy consistency of bought frozen yoghurt, but it really does taste good. If you're having it as a frozen yoghurt pot, either freeze for about 4–5 hours for a creamy dessert or overnight for a sorbet-type dessert. With the sorbet you'll need to defrost at room temperature for about half an hour.

Serves I

Fruity diet yoghurt of your choice

1. Pierce an ice lolly stick through the lid and into the centre of a yoghurt pot.
2. Freeze overnight. To remove from the pot, run the pot under hot water for a few seconds, which should be enough to loosen the sides.

Nutrition Nuggets: A great low-fat treat. If you have an ice-lolly tray, you might find you can get 2 frozen yoghurt sticks from one pot of diet yoghurt, in which case each would be counted as 0.5 GiP. Frozen yoghurt sticks or pots take much longer to eat than a pot of yoghurt and hence make you feel more satisfied.

Speedy Porridge with Grated Apple

4 GiPs per serving

Porridge has become such a convenient breakfast, all you need to do is mix raw oats with milk and pop it in the microwave on high for a couple of minutes. Rather than sweetening with sugar, this recipe uses grated apple. Choose your favourite variety of apple and add some artificial sweetener if you like. I find that UHT skimmed or semi-skimmed milk works particularly well in microwaved porridge as it becomes really creamy. So if you have some UHT cartons lying around, save them for your morning breakfast. UHT milk is just as rich in calcium as pasteurised milk. If you like your porridge thick use 30 g of oats.

Serves 1

20–30 g porridge oats, depending on thickness desired
200 ml skimmed or semi-skimmed milk
1 apple, cut into halves
Artificial sweetener, if desired

1. Mix the oats with the milk and cook in the microwave (uncovered) on high for about 2–3 minutes depending on the power of your microwave.
2. Meanwhile, grate the apple, including the skin, being careful not to go too close to the core.
3. Remove the porridge from the microwave. If it hasn't thickened, cook for another 20–30 seconds.
4. Stir in the grated apple, and artificial sweetener if desired.

Nutrition Nuggets: Porridge is a fantastic low-GI breakfast cereal. Oats help lower blood cholesterol levels. If you add honey or jam for sweetening, remember to count the GiPs.

Sautéed Bananas

1 GiP per serving

Fed up with fruit served the same old way? Then try this dish of warm, softened bananas.

Serves 1

Olive oil spray
½ banana, sliced diagonally
Lemon juice, as desired
Sprinkling of sesame seeds
Cocoa powder, to dust
Orange zest, grated

1. Heat a non-stick frying pan and add 5 sprays of oil.
2. Add the banana and sauté for a couple of minutes, adding a few drops of lemon juice to prevent sticking.
3. Serve immediately with a light sprinkling of sesame seeds, a dusting of cocoa powder and grated orange zest.

Nutrition Nuggets: Choose green-tipped bananas since they are likely to have a lower-GI rating than ripe ones.

Peaches 'n' Cream

2 GiPs per serving

You'd think this recipe would be smothered in unflavoured single or double cream, but you can creatively use some melted reduced-calorie ice cream to add a sweet and creamy touch to any fruit.

Serves 1

6 slices peaches, canned in juice
1 scoop reduced-calorie ice cream
Mint sprigs, for decoration

1. Take the ice cream out of the freezer and allow it to melt.
2. Lay the peach slices on a plate and drench in the melted ice cream. If you prefer the 'cream' to be runnier, add some of the natural juices from the canned peaches.
3. Decorate with fresh mint sprigs.

Nutrition Nuggets: When choosing canned fruit, always opt for fruit canned in water or natural juice, rather than in syrup.

Instant (Fresh) Cherry Cheesecake

1 GiP per serving

A regular cheesecake is possibly one of the most calorific desserts around, but you can eat this one with a clear, low-GI conscience. It takes about a minute to put together and is a bit of a cheating recipe, which means you spend more time eating and less time cooking!

Serves 1

1 oatcake
10 g ricotta cheese
4 cherries, stoned and halved

1. Spread the oatcake lightly with the ricotta cheese.
2. Arrange the cherries on top and serve before the oatcake goes soggy.

Nutrition Nuggets: Oatcakes offer a lower GI than standard digestive biscuit crumbs and the lower-fat ricotta cheese makes a delightful alternative to full-fat soft cheese. However, if you prefer a creamier cheese filling, then use medium-fat soft cheese (such as Light versions of cream cheese) and count this dessert as 2 GiPs per serving. Or if you fancy a different fruit, substitute the cherries with sliced peaches and count as 1.5 GiPs per serving.

Strawberry and Mint Crush

0 GiPs per serving

A refreshing drink that won't send your blood sugar soaring. You might want to add a little cold water to the blender or perhaps some sparkling water to the finished drink if you prefer a bit of fizz.

Serves 1

12 strawberries, hulled
10 fresh mint leaves
4 ice cubes

1. Simply blitz everything together in a blender and dilute with soda water, still water or sparkling water if desired.

Nutrition Nuggets: Strawberries in this quantity are GiP-free so you can enjoy this drink with a clear conscience. Fresh strawberries are rich in potassium, folate, fibre and protective antioxidants such as vitamin C.

Conversion charts

Temperature

°C	°F	Gas mark
110	225	¼
120	250	½
140	275	1
150	300	2
160	325	3
180	350	4
190	375	5
200	400	6
220	425	7
230	450	8
240	475	9

The following figures are for guidance and not intended to be precise.

Dry Measures (approx.)

28 g	1 oz
55 g	2 oz
85 g	3 oz
110 g	4 oz
225 g	8 oz
350 g	12 oz
450 g	1 lb
900 g	2 lb
1 kg	2¼ lb

Liquid Measures (approx.)

5 ml		1 tsp
15 ml		1 tbsp
25 ml	1 fl oz	5 tsp
55 ml	2 fl oz	4 tbsp
85 ml	3 fl oz	6 tbsp
115 ml	4 fl oz	8 tbsp
140 ml	5 fl oz	¼ pint
170 ml	6 fl oz	
200 ml	7 fl oz	⅓ pint
250 ml	8 fl oz	
280 ml	10 fl oz	½ pint
340 ml	12 fl oz	
420 ml	15 fl oz	¾ pint
450 ml	16 fl oz	
500 ml	18 fl oz	
570 ml	20 fl oz	1 pint
850 ml		1½ pints
1 litre		1¾ pints

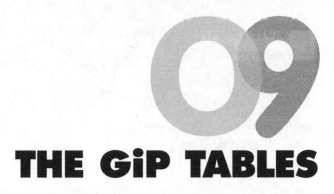

THE GiP TABLES

How to use the GiP tables

Here is your list of everyday foods with their GiP value. The tables are laid out so you can find what you need quickly. They are split into the following groups:

- ❑ Meal carbs – choose one at each meal.
- ❑ Protein – choose 2–3 portions each day.
- ❑ Vegetables.
- ❑ Fruits, desserts, snacks and drinks.
- ❑ Free flavourings.
- ❑ Meal combos that save you GiPs.
- ❑ Recipes that are low in GiPs.
- ❑ Ready meals.

There is also an alphabetical listing for quick reference – handy when you want to look up a particular food. Note that some foods in this table have been listed under their food group (e.g. cereals, soup, etc) rather than the food name, for easy GiP-comparisons. So if you can't find a particular food immediately under its own name, please look for it under the relevant category.

The guidelines

The Gi Plan works because it helps to keep you full while you lose weight, and because it is based on a balanced range of healthy foods. In order to use the tables as they are intended, follow these simple guidelines:

❑ Eat three meals and three snacks every day.

❑ Choose fruit or other low-GiP foods for snacks.

❑ Keep to the instructions alongside each group.

❑ Picture your plate in quarters and fill two quarters with vegetables (v, v), one quarter with protein (p) and one quarter with carbs (c) – remember: 'veggie, veggie, protein, carbs'.

❑ Use the serving sizes to guide you – these are designed to fill you up and help you keep a watchful eye on nutrition. If you're cooking for more than one person, use what you need to cook, but make sure what *you* eat is the portion size suggested.

❑ Use GiP-free snacks *in addition* to low-GiP snacks, not instead of them.

❑ We know that adding a low-GI food to a high one offers a reduction in the overall GI, which means your blood-

glucose levels will be more stable, and you are less likely to
feel hungry. Our healthy protein and carb meal combos
have been calculated to take this extra benefit into
account. And if you choose one of these combos you
enjoy a bonus reduction in GiPs! If you were to simply add
up the GiPs of the individual foods, you would notice that
the GiPs are lower with the combos. That's because we've
used a simple formula to take account of the benefit of
combining foods: 'high + low = medium'. Always
remember the golden rule of combining high-GiP foods
with low-GiP carbs.

☐ Look out for lower-fat or reduced-sugar versions of the
listed foods, as this will help you cut the calories.

☐ For good long-term health, keep fatty and sugary foods to
a minimum.

☐ Some ready meals have been analysed by researchers for
their GI, but this list is limited. To create low-GI culinary
delights in a dash, cast your eyes over the recipe titles in
the tables. The full recipes are given in Chapter 8.

☐ If you are a whiz in the kitchen (or even if you're not), the
GiP-free flavourings will give you a host of tempting ways
to spice up plain foods – simply adding some chilli sauce
to chick peas, or garlic to mushrooms, makes a tempting
treat in seconds. If you find other flavourings that are
virtually fat- and carb-free (check the label), go right ahead
and add them to your list.

☐ Remember the five-a-day fruit and veg mantra. The GiP-
free vegetables will help you achieve this effortlessly.

❏ You will always have a daily allowance of 200 ml (⅓ pint) of milk over and above your daily GiPs, so you can use this in drinks and in cooking without adding any extra GiPs.

❏ We have used handy household measures, so you don't necessarily have to weigh your foods. However, some weights have been given (such as 50 g dried pasta per serving). Most of the suggested serving sizes have been based on dietetic portion-size data.

❏ Note that a serving spoon is equivalent to 3 tablespoons and a teacup is an average standard teacup you would have at home.

If you have a copy of the original Gi Plan, you may notice that some of the GiP values are different. This is because we have been able to update and revise the tables as new information and data have become available.

| Food | Portion Size | Total GiPs | Special Comments |

MEAL CARBS
Choose one at each meal

BEANS AND LENTILS *(all beans and lentils count once a day as one of your five fruit and veg. These are also protein foods and if you choose them as your protein, then choose another carb)*

Food	Portion Size	Total GiPs	Special Comments
Chilli beans, canned	½ large can	1	
Haricot beans, dried, cooked	1 teacupful	1	
Lentils, red, split, dried, cooked	1 teacupful	1	
Tesco Green Lentils	½ can (150 g)	1	
Tesco Healthy Living Baked Beans	220 g can	1	
Tesco Mixed Beans Italienne	½ can (150 g)	1	
Blackeye beans, dried, cooked	1 teacupful	1.5	GI of some canned beans is not available
Butter beans, dried, cooked	1 teacupful	1.5	dried beans cook quickly in a pressure cooker
Chick peas, whole, dried, cooked	1 teacupful	1.5	
Pigeon peas, whole, dried, cooked	1 teacupful	1.5	
Pinto beans, dried, cooked	1 teacupful	1.5	
Red kidney beans, dried, cooked	1 teacupful	1.5	you can use a combination of beans in smaller portions for the same GiPs
Soya beans, dried, cooked	1 teacupful	1.5	
Baked beans, canned in tomato sauce	small can	2	
Black gram, urad gram, dried, cooked	1 teacupful	2	
Chick peas, canned	½ large can	2	great spiced up as a snack – add chilli sauce
Mung beans, whole, dried, cooked	1 teacupful	2	
Red kidney beans, canned	½ large can	2	
Chick peas, split, dried, cooked	1 teacupful	2.5	
Tesco Cannellini Beans	½ can (150 g)	2.5	
Tesco Flageolet Beans	½ can (150 g)	2.5	
Broad beans, dried, cooked	1 teacupful	3.5	

For simplicity, a teacupful is just a standard teacup you may have at home
For ease of reference, 1 serving spoon = 3 tablespoons

Food	Portion Size	Total GiPs	Special Comments
Broad beans, canned	½ large can	4	
Broad beans, frozen, cooked	1 teacupful	4	

BREADS

Food	Portion Size	Total GiPs	Special Comments
Warburtons All In One Rolls	1 roll	2	
Burgen soya and linseed bread	2 slices	2.5	grains and seeds tend to lower the GI
Sainsbury's pitta mini	1 mini pitta	2.5	
Irwin's Low GI White Bread	2 slices	2.5	contains added ingredients which lower the GI; only available in Northern Ireland at time of going to press
Barley bread	2 slices	3	
Tortilla wrap	1 wrap	3	
Granary bread	2 slices	3.5	
Mixed grain bread	2 slices	3.5	wholegrains are richer in B vitamins than refined grains
Pumpernickel bread	2 slices	3.5	
Warburtons All In One bread	2 slices	3.5	
Warburtons All In One Riddlers	1 roll	3.5	
Barley and sunflower bread	2 slices	4.5	
Chapatis, made without fat	2 small chapatis	4.5	use coarse wholemeal flour
Rye bread	2 slices	4.5	
Sainsbury's Wholemeal Pittas	1 pitta	4.5	
White bread, with added fibre	2 slices	4.5	
Hamburger buns	1 bun	5	
Pitta bread	1 pitta	5	wholemeal ones are higher in fibre
Chapatis, made with fat	2 small chapatis	5.5	
Hovis	2 slices	5.5	
White bread	2 slices	5.5	
Wholemeal bread	2 slices	5.5	opt for stoneground as it is more coarse and thus has a lower GI

For simplicity, a teacupful is just a standard teacup you may have at home
For ease of reference, 1 serving spoon = 3 tablespoons

Food	Portion Size	Total GiPs	Special Comments
Bagels, plain	1 bagel	6	a low-GiP carb filling (like sweetcorn) helps to reduce the GI of the meal
Melba toast, plain	2 toasts	7	
Taco shells, baked	1 shell	7	
Indian Pooris	2 pooris	7.5	deep fried, so have on occasion only
Baguette	1 individual	9	a great food but a very high GI. Eat always with a low-GiP carb (like salad)

BREAKFAST CEREALS (see low-combo breakfasts, page 308)

Food	Portion Size	Total GiPs	Special Comments
All Bran and semi-skimmed milk	5 tbsp + 200 ml (⅓ pint)	2	try it with sliced banana
Tesco Hi Fibre Bran Breakfast and semi-skimmed milk	30 g + 200 ml (⅓ pint)	2	
Porridge, made with water	8 tbsp of made-up porridge as per pack instructions	3	quick microwaveable breakfast. Try porridge with grated apple, see recipes
Porridge, made with milk and water	6 tbsp of made-up porridge using 100 ml (¼ pint) milk and water as required	3.5	you could try skimmed milk, 200 ml (⅓ pint), instead. Use a little sweetener, honey or fructose if you like, add the GiPs
Sainsbury's Taste the Difference Scottish jumbo oats and semi-skimmed milk	40 g + 150 ml	3.5	GI-tested on this amount, but use 30 g if you prefer it less thick
Sainsbury's wholegrain mini-wheats and semi-skimmed milk	40 g + 150 ml	3.5	GI-tested on this amount of cereal and milk
Tesco Value Muesli and semi-skimmed milk	40g + 200 ml (⅓ pint)	3.5	about 4 tbsp
Bran Flakes and semi-skimmed milk	4 tbsp + 200 ml (⅓ pint)	4	
Muesli and semi-skimmed milk	4 tbsp (40 g) + 200 ml (⅓ pint)	4	
Muesli, reduced sugar and semi-skimmed milk	4 tbsp (40 g) + 200 ml (⅓ pint)	4	

For simplicity, a teacupful is just a standard teacup you may have at home
For ease of reference, 1 serving spoon − 3 tablespoons

Food	Portion Size	Total GiPs	Special Comments
Muesli, Swiss style and semi-skimmed milk	4 tbsp (40g) + 200 ml (⅓ pint)	4	
Puffed Wheat and semi-skimmed milk	5 tbsp + 200 ml (⅓ pint)	4	a good bowl of fibre
Special K and semi-skimmed milk	5 tbsp + 200 ml (⅓ pint)	4	most cereals are enriched with vitamins
Cornflakes and semi-skimmed milk	5 tbsp + 200 ml (⅓ pint)	4.5	
Grapenuts and semi-skimmed milk	5 tbsp + 200 ml (⅓ pint)	4.5	
Instant hot oats made with semi-skimmed milk	follow pack instructions using 200 ml (⅓ pint) milk	4.5	a sachet at work could be a convenient breakfast
Nutrigrain and semi-skimmed milk	5 tbsp + 200 ml (⅓ pint)	4.5	
Raisin Splitz and semi-skimmed milk	4 tbsp + 200 ml (⅓ pint)	4.5	
Sainsbury's Precise and semi-skimmed milk	40 g + 150ml	4.5	GI-tested on this amount of cereal and milk
Shredded Wheat and semi-skimmed milk	2 biscuits + 200 ml (⅓ pint)	4.5	
Sultana Bran and semi-skimmed milk	4 tbsp + 200 ml (⅓ pint)	4.5	
Tesco Fruit & Fibre Breakfast and semi-skimmed milk	4 tbsp (40 g) + 200 ml (⅓ pint)	4.5	
Weetabix and semi-skimmed milk	2 biscuits + 200 ml (⅓ pint)	4.5	cereal for breakfast means you get calcium from milk
Rice Krispies and semi-skimmed milk	7 tbsp + 200 ml (⅓ pint)	5.5	

PASTA *(most pasta is very low in GI. Use 50 g raw per portion. Remember to add GiPs from sauces)*

Fettuccini, egg, cooked	5 tbsp (50 g dried)	1.5	try the fettuccini recipes
Spaghetti, white, cooked	50 g dried/115 g cooked	1.5	cook till *al dente* (firm to the bite)
Spaghetti, wholemeal, cooked	50 g dried/115 g cooked	1.5	try the Garlic Spaghetti recipe
Macaroni, cooked	5 tbsp (50 g dried)	2	

For simplicity, a teacupful is just a standard teacup you may have at home
For ease of reference, 1 serving spoon = 3 tablespoons

Food	Portion Size	Total GiPs	Special Comments
Noodles, instant, cooked	50 g dried/115 g cooked	2	
Linguini, thick, cooked	50 g dried/115 g cooked	2.5	make a low-fat tomato and basil sauce (page 263)
Linguini, thin, cooked	50 g dried/115 g cooked	2.5	
Egg Tagliatelle	5 tbsp (50 g dried)	3	
Noodles, rice, cooked	5 tbsp (50 g dried)	3	
Pasta, plain, cooked	5 tbsp (50 g dried)	3	
Tesco Fusilli Pasta Twists	5 tbsp (50 g dried)	3	

RICE AND GRAINS *(keep rice grains whole rather than soft and mushy)*

Food	Portion Size	Total GiPs	Special Comments
Barley, pearl, cooked	1 teacupful	1.5	throw some into soups and stews
Rice, white, Bangladeshi, boiled	2 serving spoons	1.5	available from Asian food stores
Bulgur, cooked	1 teacupful (50 g raw)	2	one of the lowest-GI grains, see recipes
Rice, brown, boiled	2 serving spoons	2.5	
Rice, white, basmati, boiled	2 serving spoons	2.5	try the Aromatic Basmati Rice recipe
Rice, white, precooked, microwaved	2 serving spoons	2.5	
Quinoa	50 g raw/170 g cooked	2.5	use instead of rice
Couscous, cooked	1 teacupful	3.5	a nice change from rice
Rice, white, easy cook, boiled	2 serving spoons	3.5	don't overcook
Rice, white, instant, boiled	2 serving spoons	3.5	
Rice, white, polished, boiled	2 serving spoons	3.5	
Rice, white, risotto, boiled	2 serving spoons	3.5	sticky rice has a higher GI so keep the grains separate
Semolina, cooked dry	1 teacupful	4.5	
Rice, white, glutinous (sticky), boiled	2 serving spoons	7	
Rice, white, jasmin, boiled	2 serving spoons	7.5	

SOUPS

Food	Portion Size	Total GiPs	Special Comments
Tomato soup, cream of, canned	1 soup bowl	1	see GiP-free Tomato Soup recipe

For simplicity, a teacupful is just a standard teacup you may have at home
For ease of reference, 1 serving spoon = 3 tablespoons

Food	Portion Size	Total GiPs	Special Comments
Instant noodle soup	1 soup bowl	2	
Lentil soup	1 soup bowl	2	wholesome and filling

STARCHY VEGETABLES *(these are part of meal carbs since they are high in starch. Other vegetables are not – you can find these on page 293)*

Food	Portion Size	Total GiPs	Special Comments
Plantain, boiled	1 plantain	1.5	choose unripe ones, available from West Indian food stores
Yam, baked	size of a medium potato	1.5	
Yam, boiled	size of a medium potato	1.5	
Yam, steamed	size of a medium potato	1.5	
Cassava, boiled	2 slices	2.5	available frozen, too
Cassava, steamed	2 slices	2.5	
Breadfruit, canned, drained	2 slices	3	
Cassava, baked	2 slices	3	frozen ones may have added fat, check labels
New potatoes, boiled	4 new potatoes	3	keep skins on
New potatoes, canned, drained	4 new potatoes	3	
Old potatoes, boiled	3 egg size potatoes	3	cold cooked potatoes have a lower GI!
Sweet potato, boiled	1 small potato	3	a source of beta-carotene
Sweet potato, steamed or microwaved	1 small potato	3	
Breadfruit, boiled	2 slices	3.5	
Sweet potato, baked	1 small potato	3.5	see recipe
Matoki, boiled	1 matoki	4	available from Asian/West Indian food stores
Chips, straight cut, frozen, oven baked	2 serving spoons	5	choose 5% fat varieties
Chips, French fries, fast food outlet	2 serving spoons	6	
Mashed potato, instant, made up with water	2 scoops	7	mashing carbs raises the GI
Old potatoes, baked	1 medium potato	7	
Parsnip, boiled	2 tbsp	7	serve with low-GiP veggies
Parsnip, roast	2 tbsp	7.5	

For simplicity, a teacupful is just a standard teacup you may have at home
For ease of reference, 1 serving spoon = 3 tablespoons

Food	Portion Size	Total GiPs	Special Comments

PROTEIN
Choose 2–3 portions a day

BEANS AND LENTILS *(all beans and lentils count once a day as one of your five fruit and veg)*

Food	Portion Size	Total GiPs	Special Comments
Chilli beans, canned	½ large can	1	
Haricot beans, dried, cooked	1 teacupful	1	
Lentils, red, split, dried, cooked	1 teacupful	1	
Tesco Green Lentils	½ can (150 g)	1	try the dahl recipes
Tesco Healthy Living Baked Beans	220 g can	1	
Tesco Mixed Beans Italienne	½ can (150 g)	1	
Tofu, cooked	150g	1	made from healthy soya beans but no fibre
Blackeye beans, dried, cooked	1 teacupful	1.5	
Butter beans, dried, cooked	1 teacupful	1.5	
Chick peas, whole, dried, cooked	1 teacupful	1.5	
Pigeon peas, whole, dried, cooked	1 teacupful	1.5	
Pinto beans, dried, cooked	1 teacupful	1.5	a low-GI wonder food
Red kidney beans, dried, cooked	1 teacupful	1.5	you can use a combination of beans in smaller portions for the same GiPs
Soya beans, dried, cooked	1 teacupful	1.5	
Baked beans, canned in tomato sauce	small can	2	
Black gram, urad gram, dried, cooked	1 teacupful	2	
Chick peas, canned	½ large can	2	great spiced up as a snack – add chilli sauce and lemon
Hummus, half-fat	¼ pot, 2 tbsp	2	
Mung beans, whole, dried, cooked	1 teacupful	2	
Peas, fresh, steamed	3 tbsp	2	
Peas, frozen, steamed	3 tbsp	2	
Red kidney beans, canned	½ large can	2	
Chick peas, split, dried, cooked	1 teacupful	2.5	
Tesco Cannellini Beans	½ can (150 g)	2.5	

For simplicity, a teacupful is just a standard teacup you may have at home
For ease of reference, 1 serving spoon = 3 tablespoons

Food	Portion Size	Total GiPs	Special Comments
Tesco Flageolet Beans	½ can (150 g)	2.5	throw beans into soups and stews
Broad beans, dried, cooked	1 teacupful	3.5	
Broad beans, canned	½ large can	4	great with red onion
Broad beans, frozen, cooked	1 teacupful	4	

EGGS *(max 5–6 per week, try omega-3 types)*

Food	Portion Size	Total GiPs	Special Comments
Eggs, boiled	2 eggs	1.5	
Eggs, fried	1 egg	1.5	or use 10 sprays of oil and count as boiled
Eggs, poached	2 eggs	1.5	
Eggs, scrambled, with milk and 1 tsp oil	2 eggs	3	
Omelette, plain, made with 1 tsp oil	2 eggs	3	

FISH *(choose fish twice a week, one being oily fish which is rich in omega-3 fats)*

Food	Portion Size	Total GiPs	Special Comments
Cockles	6 cockles	1	
Cod, baked	1 fillet	1	try the Lemony Cod recipe
Cod, grilled	1 fillet	1	
Haddock, steamed or grilled	1 fillet	1	
Lemon sole, steamed or grilled	1 fillet	1	
Oysters	1 dozen oysters	1	shellfish are a good source of zinc, great for immune function
Plaice, steamed or grilled	1 fillet	1	
Prawns	1 small jar (125 g)	1	choose fat-free dressing
Shrimps, canned in brine, drained	1 small can	1	
Tuna, canned in brine, drained	1 small can	1	half the calories of canned in oil
Crab	2 tbsp crab meat	1.5	
Haddock, smoked	1 fillet	1.5	smoked foods are higher in salt, so limit amounts
Halibut, steamed or grilled	1 fillet	1.5	
Lobster	2 tbsp	1.5	flavour with lemon juice
Mussels	6 mussels	1.5	

For simplicity, a teacupful is just a standard teacup you may have at home
For ease of reference, 1 serving spoon = 3 tablespoons

Food	Portion Size	Total GiPs	Special Comments
Salmon, smoked	3 slices	1.5	a source of healthy omega-3 fats
Scallops, steamed	3 tbsp	1.5	
Shrimps	1 teacupful	1.5	
Trout, steamed or grilled	1 fish	1.5	try the Thai-style Trout recipe
Fish fingers, cod, grilled	4 fingers	2	or freeze your own cod strips and coat with egg white
Herring, grilled	2 fillets	2	a source of healthy omega-3 fats
Salmon, pink, canned in brine, drained	small can	2	a source of healthy omega-3 fats
Salmon, steamed or grilled	1 steak	2	try Chargrilled Salmon (page 136)
Sardines, canned in brine, drained	4 sardines	2	a source of healthy omega-3 fats
Kipper, baked	2 fillets	2.5	a source of healthy omega-3 fats, but high in salt
Mackerel, canned in brine, drained	1 small can	2.5	a source of healthy omega-3 fats

MEATS

Food	Portion Size	Total GiPs	Special Comments
Beef stew, made with lean beef	2 serving spoons	1.5	limit or avoid fat in cooking
Ham	2 slices	1.5	
Kidney, ox, stewed	3 tbsp	1.5	
Lamb, loin chops, grilled, lean	2 chops	1.5	
Lamb, scrag and neck, lean only, stewed	2 serving spoons	1.5	limit or avoid fat in cooking
Rabbit, stewed	2 serving spoons	1.5	
Bacon, gammon joint, lean only, cooked	140 g steak	2	cooked weight, high in salt, limit amounts
Beef sirloin joint, roasted lean	3 slices	2	
Beef, rump steak, lean, grilled	140 g steak	2	cooked weight
Chicken, breast chunks or strips	2 serving spoons	2	

For simplicity, a teacupful is just a standard teacup you may have at home
For ease of reference, 1 serving spoon = 3 tablespoons

Food	Portion Size	Total GiPs	Special Comments
Chicken, breast, skinless, roasted	1 medium	2	
Chicken, drumstick, skinless, roasted	2 drumsticks	2	higher in fat than chicken breast
Chicken, leg, skinless, roasted	1 medium	2	
Chicken, roasted	3 slices	2	avoid the skin, breast pieces are lower in fat
Chicken, thigh, skinless, roasted	1 medium	2	
Chicken, wing, skinless, roasted	4 wings	2	
Duck, roasted	3 slices	2	avoid the skin
Kidney, lamb, sautéed	2 kidneys	2	
Liver, ox, stewed	3 tbsp	2	rich in iron and vitamin B^{12}
Pork leg joint, roasted	3 slices	2	
Pork, loin chops, grilled, lean	1 chop	2	
Turkey, roasted	2 slices	2	you get three times as much if you use wafer-thin turkey
Beef, mince, stewed	2 serving spoons	2.5	choose lean beef
Beef, topside, roasted well-done, lean	3 slices	2.5	
Corned beef, canned	2 slices	2.5	watch the salt!
Lamb, leg joint, roasted, lean	3 slices	2.5	
Lamb, shoulder joint, roasted, lean	3 slices	2.5	
Liver sausage	1 slice	2.5	all sausages tend to be high in salt and very processed
Liver, lamb, sautéed	2 slices	2.5	rich in iron, great for the immune system
Oxtail, stewed	2 serving spoons	2.5	
Tongue, ox, stewed	2 slices	2.5	
Veal, cutlet, sautéed	1 cutlet	2.5	use olive oil spray
Veal, fillet, roast	1 fillet	2.5	
Bacon rashers, back, grilled	3 rashers	3	GI of turkey rashers is not available, but they are a lower-fat choice
Beef sausages, grilled	2 sausages	3	GI of lower-fat sausages is not available, but they are a better choice

For simplicity, a teacupful is just a standard teacup you may have at home
For ease of reference, 1 serving spoon = 3 tablespoons

Food	Portion Size	Total GiPs	Special Comments
Lamb, breast, roasted, lean	3 slices	3	
Pork sausages, grilled	2 sausages	3	
Bacon rashers, middle, grilled	3 rashers	3.5	
Beefburgers, chilled/frozen, grilled	2 beefburger	3.5	
Chicken nuggets	6 nuggets	4	bake your own with chicken breast, spices and olive oil spray. Coat in egg white

MILK AND DAIRY

Food	Portion Size	Total GiPs	Special Comments
Milk, semi-skimmed	200 ml (⅓ pint)	0.5	
Milk, skimmed	200 ml (⅓ pint)	0.5	
Soya, non-dairy alternative to milk, unsweetened	200 ml (⅓ pint)	0.5	soya protein is rich in phytochemicals, shown to reduce blood cholesterol
Tesco Yoghurt Healthy Living Light Peach & Apricot	200g	0.5	
Tesco Yoghurt Healthy Living Light Strawberry	200g	0.5	
Cheese, cottage, plain, reduced fat	small tub	1	
Custard made with semi-skimmed milk	small yoghurt-pot size	1	
Drinking yoghurt	200 ml (⅓ pint)	1	choose reduced calorie if available
Flavoured milk, chocolate, reduced fat	200 ml (⅓ pint)	1	
Tesco Probiotic Original Drink	100 ml	1	
Strawberry Nesquik made with semi-skimmed milk	200 ml (⅓ pint)	1	GI has been analysed on this brand, but you can choose any brand if you like
Yoghurt, low-fat Greek style natural	150 ml	1	
Yoghurt, Greek, Sheep's	150 ml	1	
Yoghurt, low-fat, natural	small pot	1	
Cheese, Ricotta	small tub (150 g)	1.5	fantastic low-fat option

For simplicity, a teacupful is just a standard teacup you may have at home
For ease of reference, 1 serving spoon = 3 tablespoons

Food	Portion Size	Total GiPs	Special Comments
Cheese, cottage, plain	small tub	1.5	
Fromage frais, virtually fat-free	150 ml pot	1.5	
Ice cream, reduced-calorie	1 scoop	1.5	add some lemon zest for zing
Cheese, soft, medium-fat, (e.g. light version of cream cheese)	25 g	2	if you use extra light, have a little more
Chocolate Nesquik made with semi-skimmed milk	200 ml (⅓ pint)	2	
Crème fraîche, half fat	50 ml	2	watch portion size
Cheese, Edam	matchbox-size piece (25 g)	2.5	
Cheese, Feta	matchbox-size piece (25 g)	2.5	
Cheese, Mini Babybel Light	1 individual portion	2.5	
Cheese, Camembert	matchbox-size piece (25 g)	3	lower in fat than Brie
Cheese, Cheddar, half-fat	matchbox-size piece (25 g)	3	
Cheese, Mozzarella	matchbox-size piece (25 g)	3	
Cheese, Brie	matchbox-size piece (25 g)	3.5	
Cheese, Cheshire	matchbox-size piece (25 g)	4	
Cheese, Emmental	matchbox-size piece (25 g)	4	
Cheese, Blue Stilton	matchbox-size piece (25 g)	4.5	
Cheese, Cheddar	matchbox-size piece (25 g)	4.5	grated goes further, use 3 tbsp

NUTS *(use nuts in cooking to provide protein)*

Food	Portion Size	Total GiPs	Special Comments
Almonds	10–12 almonds	3	high in fat but low in GI and saturates, choose nuts once a day strictly in these amounts
Peanuts, dry roasted	pub pack (25 g) or half 50 g pack	3	high in fat but low in saturates and GI, choose nuts once a day strictly in these amounts

For simplicity, a teacupful is just a standard teacup you may have at home
For ease of reference, 1 serving spoon = 3 tablespoons

Food	Portion Size	Total GiPs	Special Comments
Peanuts, in shells	15 shells	3	shells help you limit intake and nuts are unsalted
Peanuts, roasted and salted	pub pack (25 g) or half 50 g pack	3	high in fat but low in saturates and GI, choose nuts once a day strictly in these amounts
Pecans	12 halves	3	choose nuts once a day stictly in these amounts
Walnuts	8 halves	3	throw them into salads, choose nuts once a day stictly in these amounts
Cashew nuts	15 cashews	3.5	high in fat but low in GI, choose nuts once a day strictly in these amounts

VEGETABLES

Packed with GiP-free choices

Alfalfa sprouts	as desired	0
Artichoke, globe	as desired	0
Asparagus	as desired	0
Asparagus, canned, drained	as desired	0
Aubergines, grilled	as desired	0
Bamboo shoots, canned, drained	as desired	0
Broccoli, green, frozen, steamed	as desired	0
Broccoli, green, raw	as desired	0
Broccoli, green, steamed	as desired	0
Broccoli, purple sprouting, steamed	as desired	0
Brussels sprouts, frozen, steamed	12 sprouts	0
Brussels sprouts, steamed	12 sprouts	0
Cabbage spring steamed	as desired	0
Cabbage winter, steamed	as desired	0
Cabbage, Chinese, raw	as desired	0
Cabbage, frozen, steamed	as desired	0

} contains iron

For simplicity, a teacupful is just a standard teacup you may have at home
For ease of reference, 1 serving spoon = 3 tablespoons

Food	Portion Size	Total GiPs	Special Comments
Cabbage, raw	as desired	0	raw is a good source of vitamin C
Cabbage, red, steamed	as desired	0	
Cabbage, Savoy, steamed	as desired	0	
Cabbage, summer, steamed	as desired	0	
Cabbage, white, steamed	as desired	0	
Cauliflower, frozen, steamed	as desired	0	
Cauliflower, raw	as desired	0	
Cauliflower, steamed	as desired	0	
Celeriac, raw	as desired	0	
Celeriac, steamed	as desired	0	
Celery, raw	as desired	0	source of potassium
Celery, steamed	as desired	0	
Chard, Swiss, raw	as desired	0	
Chard, Swiss, steamed	as desired	0	
Chicory, raw	as desired	0	
Chicory, steamed	as desired	0	
Courgette, cooked in spray oil	as desired	0	use 5 sprays of oil, see the recipe for Chargrilled Courgette Ribbons
Courgette, raw	as desired	0	
Courgette, steamed	as desired	0	
Cucumber, raw	as desired	0	
Curly kale, steamed	as desired	0	
Endive, raw	as desired	0	
Fennel, raw	as desired	0	
Fennel, steamed	as desired	0	
French and green beans	as desired	0	
Gherkins, pickled, drained	as desired	0	
Gourd, kantola, canned, drained	as desired	0	
Gourd, karela, canned, drained	as desired	0	
Gourd, tinda, canned, drained	as desired	0	
Kohl rabi, raw	as desired	0	

For simplicity, a teacupful is just a standard teacup you may have at home
For ease of reference, 1 serving spoon = 3 tablespoons

Food	Portion Size	Total GiPs	Special Comments
Kohl rabi, steamed	as desired	0	
Leeks, steamed	as desired	0	
Lettuce, butterhead, raw	as desired	0	
Lettuce, Cos, raw	as desired	0	
Lettuce, Iceberg, raw	as desired	0	
Lettuce, mixed leaves	as desired	0	
Lettuce, Webbs, raw	as desired	0	
Lotus tubers, canned	as desired	0	
Marrow, parwal, canned, drained	as desired	0	
Marrow, steamed	as desired	0	filling and low in calories
Mooli – see Radish, white			
Mushrooms, raw	as desired	0	
Mushrooms, canned, drained	as desired	0	
Mushrooms, oyster, raw	as desired	0	
Mushrooms, steamed	as desired	0	
Mushrooms, straw, canned, drained	as desired	0	
Mustard and cress, raw	as desired	0	
Mustard leaves, steamed	as desired	0	
Okra, canned, drained	as desired	0	
Okra, steamed	as desired	0	
Onions, cooked	as desired	0	
Onions, pickled, cocktail/silverskin, drained	as desired	0	
Pak Choi	as desired	0	great in soups (see Hot and Sour Soup recipe)
Peppers, capsicum, steamed	as desired	0	
Peppers, raw	as desired	0	rich in vitamin C
Raddiccio (salad leaves)	as desired	0	
Radish, red, raw	as desired	0	
Radish leaves	as desired	0	
Radish, white/mooli, raw	as desired	0	
Sauerkraut	as desired	0	

For simplicity, a teacupful is just a standard teacup you may have at home
For ease of reference, 1 serving spoon = 3 tablespoons

Food	Portion Size	Total GiPs	Special Comments
Seakale, steamed	as desired	0	
Shallots, raw	as desired	0	
Spinach, canned, drained	as desired	0	
Spinach, frozen, steamed	as desired	0	
Spinach, raw	as desired	0	cancer-protective
Spinach, steamed	as desired	0	
Spring greens, steamed	as desired	0	
Spring onions, bulbs and tops, raw	as desired	0	
Sweetcorn, baby, canned, drained	as desired	0	
Sweetcorn, baby, fresh and frozen, steamed	as desired	0	
Tomatoes, canned, with juice	as desired	0	rich in cancer-fighting lycopene
Tomatoes, cherry, raw	as desired	0	
Tomatoes, raw	as desired	0	make a sauce with spray oil, onion, garlic and herbs
Turnip, steamed	as desired	0	
Vine leaves, preserved in brine	as desired	0	
Watercress, raw	as desired	0	
Carrot, average raw	1 large carrot	0.5	
Carrots, fresh, steamed	2 tbsp	0.5	
Carrots, frozen, steamed	2 tbsp	0.5	
Carrots, young, steamed	2 tbsp	0.5	
Chilli beans, canned	½ large can	1	
Courgette, sautéed	1 courgette	1	or use spray oil and count as 0
Haricot beans, dried, cooked	1 teacupful	1	
Lentils, red, split, dried, cooked	1 teacupful	1	
Tesco Green Lentils	½ can (150 g)	1	try the Green Lentil Dahl recipe
Tesco Healthy Living Baked Beans	220 g can	1	
Tesco Mixed Beans Italienne	½ can (150 g)	1	
Blackeye beans, dried, cooked	1 teacupful	1.5	GI of some canned beans is not available

For simplicity, a teacupful is just a standard teacup you may have at home
For ease of reference, 1 serving spoon = 3 tablespoons

Food	Portion Size	Total GiPs	Special Comments
Butter beans, canned	½ can	1.5	
Butter beans, dried, cooked	1 teacupful	1.5	
Chick peas, whole, dried, cooked	1 teacupful	1.5	
Pigeon peas, whole, dried, cooked	1 teacupful	1.5	
Pinto beans, dried, cooked	1 teacupful	1.5	
Plantain, steamed	1 plantain	1.5	choose unripe variety
Red kidney beans, dried, cooked	1 teacupful	1.5	you can use a combination of beans in smaller portions for the same GiPs
Seaweed, nori, dried, raw	2 tbsp	1.5	contains the antioxidant selenium
Soya beans, dried, cooked	1 teacupful	1.5	
Yam, baked	size of a medium potato	1.5	
Yam, boiled	size of a medium potato	1.5	
Yam, steamed	size of a medium potato	1.5	
Ackee, canned, drained	½ can	2	
Baked beans, canned in tomato sauce	1 small can	2	
Beetroot, pickled, drained	4 slices	2	
Black gram, urad gram, dried, cooked	1 teacupful	2	
Chick peas, canned	½ large can	2	great spiced up as a snack – add chilli sauce
Mung beans, whole, dried, cooked	1 teacupful	2	
Mushrooms, common, stir-fried	2 tbsp	2	or use spray oil and have them free
Peas, fresh, steamed	3 tbsp	2	
Peas, frozen, steamed	3 tbsp	2	source of protein
Red kidney beans, canned	½ large can	2	
Sweetcorn, on-the-cob, whole, steamed or grilled	1 sweetcorn cob	2	add a little water and herbs and cook in the microwave
Beetroot, cooked	4 slices	2.5	
Cassava, boiled	size of a medium potato	2.5	you can buy cassava frozen

For simplicity, a teacupful is just a standard teacup you may have at home
For ease of reference, 1 serving spoon = 3 tablespoons

Food	Portion Size	Total GiPs	Special Comments
Cassava, steamed	size of a medium potato	2.5	
Chick peas, split, dried, cooked	1 teacupful	2.5	
Sweetcorn, kernels, canned,drained	3 tbsp	2.5	choose canned veg in unsalted, unsweetened water
Sweetcorn, kernels, fresh, cooked	3 tbsp	2.5	
Tesco Cannellini Beans	½ can (150 g)	2.5	
Tesco Flageolet Beans	½ can (150 g)	2.5	throw beans into soups and stews
Breadfruit, canned, drained	2 slices	3	
Cassava, baked	size of a medium potato	3	available frozen in some supermarkets
New potatoes, boiled	4 new potatoes	3	
New potatoes, canned, drained	4 new potatoes	3	
Old potatoes, boiled	3 egg-size potatoes	3	cold cooked potatoes have a lower GI!
Pumpkin, cooked	2 slices	3	
Swede, steamed	2 tbsp	3	
Sweet potato, boiled	1 small potato	3	
Sweet potato, steamed	1 small potato	3	
Breadfruit, boiled	2 slices	3.5	
Broad beans, boiled	2 tbsp	3.5	
Broad beans, dried, cooked	1 teacupful	3.5	
Sweet potato, baked	1 small potato	3.5	
Broad beans, canned	½ large can	4	
Broad beans, frozen, cooked	1 teacupful	4	
Matoki, boiled	1 matoki	4	
Chips, straight cut, frozen, oven baked	2 serving spoons	5	choose 5% fat versions
Chips, French fries, fast food outlet	2 serving spoons	6	
Instant mashed potato made up with water	2 scoops	7	use the same GiP for homemade, add any GiPs from milk or butter
Old potatoes, baked	1 medium potato	7	
Parsnip, steamed	2 tbsp	7	a great veg, but high in GI
Parsnip, roast	2 tbsp	7.5	

For simplicity, a teacupful is just a standard teacup you may have at home
For ease of reference, 1 serving spoon = 3 tablespoons

| Food | Portion Size | Total GiPs | Special Comments |

FRUITS, DESSERTS, SNACKS, DRINKS

Fruit gets the gold star

BAKERY

Food	Portion Size	Total GiPs	Special Comments
Crumpets	1 crumpet	4	
Currant bread (fruit loaf)	2 slices	4	no butter please!
Currant bun	1 bun	4	
Banana bread	1 slice	4.5	
Scotch pancakes	2 pancakes	5	
Melba toast, plain	2 toast	7	
Scone, plain	1 scone	10	very high GI, hence high GiPs value

BISCUITS

Food	Portion Size	Total GiPs	Special Comments
Oat cakes	1 oat cake	1	oats are low GI
Jacob Essentials – Wholewheat crackers with sesame seeds & rosemary	2 triangles	2	or have one for 1 GiP
Rich tea	2 biscuits	2	
Cream crackers	2 crackers	3	
Crispbread, rye	2 crispbread	3	
Ryvita	2 crispbread	3	
Wholemeal crackers	2 crackers	3	
Rice cakes	2 cakes	7	calories per rice cake are low, but GI is high
Water biscuits	2 biscuits	7.5	calories per biscuit are low, but GI is high

DRINKS

Food	Portion Size	Total GiPs	Special Comments
Coffee, no sugar	as desired	0	use milk from allowance
Diet soft drinks	as desired	0	you could go for decaff versions
Sugar-free squash	as desired	0	freeze into an ice-lolly for a change

For simplicity, a teacupful is just a standard teacup you may have at home
For ease of reference, 1 serving spoon = 3 tablespoons

Food	Portion Size	Total GiPs	Special Comments
Tea, no sugar	as desired	0	use milk from allowance
Tomato juice	1 glass (150 ml)	0	add some Worcester sauce for a bit of zing!
Water, sparkling	as desired	0	
Water, still	as desired	0	
Water, sugar-free flavoured	as desired	0	check no added sugar
Apple juice, unsweetened	1 glass (150 ml)	1	keep to portion size, cloudy has a slightly lower GI
Vie Shot Apple/Carrot/Strawberry	100 ml	1	other flavours may have a different GI
Grapefruit juice, unsweetened	1 glass (150 ml)	1.5	
innocent kids Oranges, Mangoes and Pineapples	180 ml carton	1.5	keep to portion size
Orange juice, unsweetened	1 glass (150 ml)	1.5	
Pineapple juice, unsweetened	1 glass (150 ml)	1.5	
innocent Mangoes and Passionfruit	1 glass (150 ml)	2	pour this amount from a litre pack
innocent Strawberries and Bananas	1 glass (150 ml)	2	pour this amount from a litre pack
Vie Shot Orange/Banana/Carrot	100 ml	2	other flavours may have a different GI
Cranberry juice	1 glass (150 ml)	3	diet versions are lower in calories, but GI value is not available

FRUIT *(have five fruit and veg a day: they're rich in antioxidants)*

Grapefruit	1 grapefruit	0	rich in potassium which helps to regulate blood pressure
Raspberries	1 teacupful	0	keep to portion size if you want to have them GiP-free
Strawberries	1 teacupful or 12	0	try the Strawberry and Mint Crush recipe
Apples	1 apple	0.5	the whole fruit has all the fibre, choose it over fruit juice
Cherries	12 cherries	0.5	
Kiwi fruit	1 kiwi	0.5	abundant in vitamin C

For simplicity, a teacupful is just a standard teacup you may have at home
For ease of reference, 1 serving spoon = 3 tablespoons

Food	Portion Size	Total GiPs	Special Comments
Olives	10 olives	0.5	olives with stones take longer to eat so you might eat less
Peaches, canned in juice	6 slices	0.5	
Pears	1 pear	0.5	
Plums	3 plums	0.5	
Fruit cocktail, canned in juice	½ large can	1	
Raisins	1 tbsp	1	
Oranges	1 large orange	1.5	the GI of satsumas is not available, but you can choose 2–3 satsumas instead of an orange and count the GiPs as 1.5
Peaches	1 peach	1.5	
Pears, canned in juice	2 pear halves	1.5	
Prunes, ready-to-eat	8 prunes	1.5	
Apricots, dried	4 apricots	2	good source of fibre and beta-carotene
Avocado	1 small avocado	2	
Bananas	1 small banana	2	great source of potassium
Custard apple	1 custard apple	2	
Dates, dried	4 dates	2	
Grapes	15 grapes	2	
Mangoes	1 small mango	2	try the Mango Smoothie recipe
Melon, cantaloupe	½ melon	2	
Apricots, fresh	4 apricots	2.5	
Paw-paw	½ small	2.5	
Pineapple	1 slice	2.5	
Figs, dried	2 figs	3	
Sultanas	2 handfuls	3	count 1 tbsp as 1 GiP
Melon, watermelon	1 slice	3.5	

MILK AND DAIRY

Milk, semi-skimmed	200 ml (⅓ pint)	0.5	
Milk, skimmed	200 ml (⅓ pint)	0.5	

For simplicity, a teacupful is just a standard teacup you may have at home
For ease of reference, 1 serving spoon = 3 tablespoons

Food	Portion Size	Total GiPs	Special Comments
Soya, non-dairy alternative to milk, unsweetened	200 ml (⅓ pint)	0.5	soya protein is rich in phytochemicals, shown to reduce blood cholesterol
Tesco Yoghurt Healthy Living Light Peach & Apricot	200 g	0.5	
Tesco Yoghurt Healthy Living Light Strawberry	200 g	0.5	
Custard made with semi-skimmed milk	small yoghurt-pot size	1	
Drinking yoghurt	200 ml (⅓ pint)	1	choose reduced-calorie if available
Flavoured milk, chocolate, reduced fat	200 ml (⅓ pint)	1	
Strawberry Nesquik made with semi-skimmed milk	200 ml (⅓ pint)	1	GI has been analysed on this brand, but you can choose any brand if you like
Tesco Probiotic Original Drink	100 ml	1	
Tzatziki	2 tbsp	1	opt for lower-fat versions if available
Yoghurt, low-fat Greek style natural	150 ml	1	
Yoghurt, diet	1 small pot	1	
Yoghurt, Greek, Sheep's	150 ml	1	
Yoghurt, low-fat, natural	small pot	1	
Fromage frais, virtually fat free	150 ml pot	1.5	
Ice cream, reduced-calorie	1 scoop	1.5	
Mousse, reduced-fat	1 small pot	1.5	
Ice cream, dairy, vanilla	1 scoop	2	try frozen yoghurt instead
Chocolate Nesquik made with semi-skimmed milk	200 ml (⅓ pint)	2	
Soya, alternative to yogurt, fruit	1 small pot	2	

SNACKS (nuts in shells take longer to eat, so you may end up having less)

Sesame seeds	2 tsp	1	throw them into GiP-free salad for extra crunch

For simplicity, a teacupful is just a standard teacup you may have at home
For ease of reference, 1 serving spoon = 3 tablespoons

Food	Portion Size	Total GiPs	Special Comments
Almonds	10–12 almonds	3	high in fat but low in GI and saturates, choose nuts once a day strictly in these amounts
Peanuts, dry roasted	pub pack (25 g) or half 50 g pack	3	high in fat but low in GI and saturates, choose nuts once a day strictly in these amounts
Peanuts, roasted and salted	pub pack (25 g) or half 50 g pack	3	high in fat but low in GI and saturates, choose nuts once a day strictly in these amounts
Pecan nuts	12 halves	3	choose nuts once a day stictly in these amounts
Walnuts	8 halves	3	high in fat but low in GI and saturates, choose nuts once a day strictly in these amounts
GoLower Nut Bar – Coconut	1 bar (34 g)	3	no extra nuts on same day
GoLower Nut Bar – Chocolate	1 bar (34 g)	3	no extra nuts on same day
GoLower Nut Bar – Raspberry	1 bar (34 g)	3	no extra nuts on same day
Bright Bar Energise	1 bar (35 g)	3.5	
Bright Bar Inside	1 bar (35 g)	3.5	
Cashew nuts	15 cashews	3.5	high in fat but low in GI, choose nuts once a day strictly in these amounts
Popcorn, plain	5 tbsp	4	choose lower-fat varieties, or make your own
Cereal chewy bar – dried fruit	45–50 g bar	4.5	
Cereal crunchy bar – dried fruit	45–50 g bar	4.5	
Pretzels	25 g portion	6	a low-fat snack but high in GI

SOUPS

Food	Portion Size	Total GiPs	Special Comments
Minestrone soup, dried, as served	1 soup bowl	0	GI of only these packet soups is available, but you can try other flavours

For simplicity, a teacupful is just a standard teacup you may have at home
For ease of reference, 1 serving spoon = 3 tablespoons

Food	Portion Size	Total GiPs	Special Comments
Tomato soup, dried, as served	1 soup bowl	0.5	
Tomato soup, cream of, canned	1 soup bowl	1	
Instant noodle soup	1 soup bowl	2	
Lentil soup	1 soup bowl	2	or try the Lentil and Coriander Soup recipe (1 GiP)

FREE FLAVOURINGS
(Choose as often as you like)

Artificial sweeteners		0	if you have a lot, vary the types
Chilli sauce		0	
Dressing, fat-free		0	limit to about 2 tbsp
Herbs, fresh or dried		0	
Jelly, sugar-free	as desired	0	
Mustard, any type		0	
Oil, spray oil		0	up to 10 sprays per dish, strict portion limit
Pepper, any type		0	
Salt		0	keep added salt to a minimum
Salt substitutes		0	about ⅔ less sodium than salt
Soy sauce		0	try low-sodium types
Spices fresh (eg. garlic, ginger, chilli)		0	use crushed in jars for convenience
Spices ground (eg. paprika, chilli powder, curry powder)		0	try the Cajun-spiced Turkey recipe
Spices whole (eg. cumin seeds, coriander seeds, caraway seeds)		0	
Stock cube or bouillon		0	try low-sodium types
Tomato purée		0	
Vinegar (rice, balsamic, malt, wine)		0	try the Hot and Sour Soup recipe
Worcester sauce		0	

For simplicity, a teacupful is just a standard teacup you may have at home
For ease of reference, 1 serving spoon = 3 tablespoons

Food	Portion Size	Total GiPs	Special Comments

FATTY AND SUGARY FOODS

Keep to a minimum

CAKES AND BISCUITS

Food	Portion Size	Total GiPs	Special Comments
Digestive biscuits, plain	1 biscuit	3.5	reduced-fat versions are available
Muffins, American style, chocolate chip	1 muffin	5	choosing a smaller one means fewer calories
Muffins, blueberry	1 muffin	5	
Muffins, oat bran	1 muffin	5	
Scotch pancakes	2 pancakes	5	
Danish pastries	small pastry	5.5	pastry is often rich in trans fats
Croissants	1 croissant	6	
Sponge cake	small slice	6	watch portion size
Waffles	1 waffle	6.5	
Doughnuts, ring	1 doughnut	7.5	
Shortbread	2 fingers	7.5	

FATS AND OILS *(opt for monounsaturated ones)*

Food	Portion Size	Total GiPs	Special Comments
Spray oil	up to 10 sprays per dish	0	
Spread, half-fat, unsaturated	scraping	0.5	some are monounsaturated
Spread, low-fat	scraping	0.5	
Spread, very low-fat, unsaturated	1 tsp	0.5	
Butter	scraping	1	
Spread, half-fat, unsaturated	1 tsp	1	
Spread, low-fat	1 tsp	1	
Oil, olive oil	1 tsp	1.5	monounsaturated
Oil, rapeseed oil	1 tsp	1.5	monounsaturated; also sometimes sold as vegetable oil – check label
Butter	1 tsp	2	

For simplicity, a teacupful is just a standard teacup you may have at home
For ease of reference, 1 serving spoon = 3 tablespoons

Food	Portion Size	Total GiPs	Special Comments
Oil, sunflower oil	1 tsp	2	if cooking for 4, use 4 tsp and then count your portion as 2 GiPs
Oil, vegetable oil, mixed	1 tsp	2	
Mayonnaise, reduced calorie	1 tbsp	3	or count 1 tsp as 1 GiP

PROCESSED FOODS

Food	Portion Size	Total GiPs	Special Comments
Bacon rashers, back, grilled	3 rashers	3	GI of turkey rashers is not available, but they are a lower-fat choice
Beef sausages, grilled	2 sausages	3	GI of lower-fat sausages is not available, but they are a better choice
Pork sausages, grilled	2 sausages	3	
Bacon rashers, middle, grilled	3 rashers	3.5	
Beefburgers, chilled/frozen, grilled	2 beefburgers	3.5	try the Beefier Burgers recipe
Pizza, cheese and tomato, deep pan	2 slices from medium (9" diameter) or 1 slice of large (12" diameter)	3.5	GI of other pizza toppings not available – if choosing meat toppings, opt for lower-fat types
Pizza, cheese and tomato, thin base	2 slices from medium (9" diameter) or 1 slice of large (12" diameter)	3.5	GI of other pizza toppings not available – if choosing meat toppings – avoid extra cheese
Pizza, vegetarian	2 slices from medium (9" diameter) or 1 slice of large (12" diameter)	3.5	choose less cheese and more veggies
Chicken nuggets, take-away	6 nuggets	4	high in salt
Cornish pasty	1 pasty	4	pastry is high in fat
Steak and kidney/Beef pie, individual, chilled/frozen, baked	1 pie	4.5	
Chips, straight cut, frozen, oven baked	2 serving spoons	5	thicker chips absorb less fat
Chips, French fries, fast food outlet	2 serving spoons	6	
Taco shells, baked	1 shell	7	try the Crispy Tortilla Chips recipe

For simplicity, a teacupful is just a standard teacup you may have at home
For ease of reference, 1 serving spoon = 3 tablespoons

Food	Portion Size	Total GiPs	Special Comments
Indian Pooris	2 pooris	7.5	deep-fried, watch out!

CRISPS

Corn chips	small packet (30 g)	6	try the 3-GiP Crispy Tortilla Chips recipe
Potato crisps	small packet (25 g)	6.5	

SUGARY FOODS *(see also nut and cereal bars, page 303)*

Jam, reduced sugar	1 tsp	0.5	
Marmalade, reduced sugar	1 tsp	0.5	
Fructose	2 tsp	1	
Honey	1 tsp	1	
Jam	1 tsp	1	
Marmalade	1 tsp	1	
Chocolate, milk	1 square piece	1.5	
Chocolate, milk	1 treat-size bar (15 g)	2	
Chocolate, white	1 treat-size bar (13 g)	2	
Snickers bar	1 fun size (19 g)	2	
Sugar	2 tsp	2.5	
Twix	1 mini Twix (21 g)	2.5	
Mars bar	1 fun size (19 g)	3	
Jellybeans	6 jelly beans	4	
Nougat	4 sweets	4	
Chocolate-covered peanuts (e.g. M&M)	1 small pack (47 g)	5	
Sparkling glucose drink	1 glass (150 ml)	7	
Glucose – liquid	2 tsp	9.5	goes straight into the bloodstream!

For simplicity, a teacupful is just a standard teacup you may have at home
For ease of reference, 1 serving spoon = 3 tablespoons

Food	Portion Size	Total GiPs	Special Comments

GO LOW WITH A COMBO

Made-up healthy choices that can save you GiPs.
You could add a fruit or fruit juice to provide balance.

BREAKFAST CHOICES *(see also Breakfast Cereals, page 283)*

Food	Total GiPs	Special Comments
Oat cakes (2) with low-fat spread (scraping) and plain cottage cheese (small tub)	2.5	
Peanut butter (2 tsp) on 1 slice of wholemeal bread	3.5	no nuts allowed on the same day.; GI for peanut butter on its own is not available
Granary bread (2 slices) with scrambled egg (2) and tomato	6	

LUNCH AND DINNER CHOICES

Food	Total GiPs	Special Comments
Burgen Soya and linseed bread (2 slices) with low-fat spread (1 tsp), tuna (small can, in brine, drained) and cucumber	3	
Burgen soya and linseed bread (2 slices) with low-fat spread (scraping) and Edam cheese (small matchbox-size piece)	4	
Tortilla wrap (1) with chicken (3 slices) and mixed green salad	4	wholemeal tortilla has more fibre
Tortilla wrap (1) with mozzarella cheese (small matchbox size-piece, chopped), beef tomato and basil	4.5	
Granary bread (2 slices) with low-fat spread (1 tsp), ham (2 slices) and salad	5	or use mustard (coarse-grain or spread) instead of low-fat spread
Granary bread (2 slices) with low-fat spread (1 tsp), mozzarella cheese (1 slice) fresh basil and tomato	5.5	
Pumpernickel bread (2 slices) and low-fat spread (1 tsp), ham (2 slices), mixed green salad	5.5	
Wholemeal bread (2 slices) with low-fat spread (scraping) and banana (1)	6	seeded breads are lower GI
Jacket potato with low-fat spread (1 tsp), cottage cheese (small tub) and sliced peppers	6.5	

For simplicity, a teacupful is just a standard teacup you may have at home
For ease of reference, 1 serving spoon = 3 tablespoons

Food	Portion Size	Total GiPs	Special Comments
Wholemeal bread (2 slices) with low-fat spread (1 tsp), cottage cheese (small tub) and shredded cucumber and lettuce		6.5	
Jacket potato with low-fat spread (1 tsp), tuna (small can, in brine, drained) and sweetcorn (3 tbsp)		7	sweetcorn helps lower the GI
Wholemeal bread (2 slices) with low-fat spread (1 tsp), melted Edam (1 thin slice) and tomato		7	
Wholemeal bread (2 slices) with butter (1 tsp) and poached eggs (2)		8	
Jacket potato with low-fat spread (1 tsp), half-fat Cheddar cheese (3 tbsp grated) and side salad (fat-free dressing)		9.5	grated cheese goes further
Baguette (1 small) with low-fat spread (1 tsp), prawns (125 g) and mixed green salad (fat-free dressing)		10.5	
Baguette (1 small) with low-fat spread (1 tsp), roast beef (3 slices), lettuce and mustard		12	

For more Lunch and Dinner Choices see recipes below

THE RECIPES

See Chapter 8

All GiPs in the recipes are per serving

SOUPS, STARTERS AND SIDES

Chargrilled Courgette Ribbons	0	takes about 5 minutes
Chilled Gazpacho	0	great on a warm summer's day
Chilli and Lime Rocket Leaves	0	
Creamed Aubergine with Garlic	0	
Coriander Chutney	0	
Hot and Sour Soup	0	
Lemony Chestnut Mushrooms	0	you can use any mushrooms
Mixed Pepper Salsa	0	a good way to get vitamin C
Roasted Mediterranean Vegetables	0	

For simplicity, a teacupful is just a standard teacup you may have at home
For ease of reference, 1 serving spoon = 3 tablespoons

Food	Portion Size	Total GiPs	Special Comments
Speedy Salsa Sauce		0	
Stir-fried Crunchy Vegetables		0	
Tomato Soup with Crunchy Onions and Green Pepper 'Croutons'		0	takes 10 minutes to make
Tomato and Mustard Seed Salad		0	
Veg Box		0	keep one in fridge
Warming Marrow and Leek Soup		0	
Wheat-free Tabbouleh		0	
Caramelised Carrots		0.5	
Olive and Cucumber Snack Box		0.5	keep one at work
Cheat's Whole Lentil and Coriander Soup		1	uses canned lentils
Marmalade Chutney		1	
Rustic Red Lentil and Basil Soup		1	freezes well
Speedy Cucumber and Mint Raita		1	
Spicy Baked Beans		1	takes less than a minute
Farmhouse Barley and Lentil broth		2	
Middle-Eastern Tabbouleh		2	
Simple Bulgur Wheat		2	for a spicy version, see the Lemony Cod Strips recipe
Stir-fried Noodles with Crispy Vegetables		2	
Aromatic Basmati Rice		2.5	
Crispy Tortilla Chips		3	great with spicy salsa
Roasted Sweet Potato Slices		3	

MEAT AND POULTRY

Food	Portion Size	Total GiPs	Special Comments
Juicy Drumsticks with Roasted Shallots		2	
Minty Lamb Chops on Roasted Apple Rings		2	
Chilli Chicken on Granary		2.5	
Turkey (or Chicken) and Almond Koftas with Warm Plum Chutney		2.5	
Beefier Burgers		3	choose a granary or low-GI bun
Citrus Roast Chicken Parcels		3	
Pan-fried Turkey Breasts with Cajun Spice and Tarragon		3.5	

For simplicity, a teacupful is just a standard teacup you may have at home
For ease of reference, 1 serving spoon = 3 tablespoons

Food	Portion Size	Total GiPs	Special Comments
Beef Chow Mein		4	
Chicken Fajitas		4	great for using leftovers
Creamy Tagliatelli with Ham and Field Mushrooms		4	
Chilli Con Carne		4.5	

FISH

Tandoori Prawns		1.5	
Thai-style Trout with Basil and Ginger		1.5	
Tuna (or Egg) Niçoise		2	
Sesame Prawn Toasts		2.5	
Stuffed Mackerel		2.5	
Lemony Cod Strips with Spicy Bulgur Wheat		3	
Tuna Pasta Salad		4	
Potato, Apple and Tuna Salad		4.5	

VEGETABLE MAINS

10-minute Mushroom Stroganoff		1	
Green Lentil Dahl		1	
Red Lentil Dahl with Lime and Coriander		1	
Quorn and Chick Pea Curry		2	
Baked Flat Mushrooms with Melted Camembert		3	
Garlic Spaghetti with Courgette Ribbons		3	
Greek Salad		3	
Fettuccine with Creamy Spinach Sauce and Marinated Tomatoes		3.5	vibrant colours, and packed with nutrients
Creamy Tagliatelli with Chilli Beans and Field Mushrooms		4	if you use fettucinne or spaghetti count as 3 GiPs
Main Meal Dahl and Peanut Soup		4	
Spinach and Ricotta Cannelloni		4	seriously tasty
Vegetable Pasta in Rich Tomato and Basil Sauce		4.5	use this sauce for any pasta
Nutty Couscous with Lime and Parsley		5	no nuts on the same day
Savoury French Toast		5	

For simplicity, a teacupful is just a standard teacup you may have at home
For ease of reference, 1 serving spoon = 3 tablespoons

Food	Portion Size	Total GiPs	Special Comments

SWEET THINGS

Food	Portion Size	Total GiPs	Special Comments
Strawberry and Mint Crush		0	
Frozen Yoghurt Sticks		1	a long-lasting, satisfying treat
Instant (Fresh) Cherry Cheesecake		1	
Sautéed Bananas		1	warming and comforting
Spiced Pear with Ginger Fromage Frais		1	
Mango Smoothie		2	filling and delicious
Peaches 'n' Cream		2	
Speedy Porridge with Grated Apple		4	

READY MEALS

Food	Portion Size	Total GiPs	Special Comments
Instant gravy	2 serving spoons	0.5	can be high in salt, but lower in fat than using meat juices
Quorn, pieces, as purchased	12 pieces	1	a great low-fat meat substitute, use the same GiP as two Quorn burgers
Ravioli, meat	12 ravioli	1.5	
Dhokra, Indian	4 pieces	2	
Tesco Roasted Winter Vegetables	200 g (½ pack)	2	
Sushi	6 mini	2.5	
Tesco Mushroom burger	87.5 g (½ pack)	2.5	grill to keep the fat down
Sainsbury's Be Good to Yourself Egg & Cress Sandwich	per pack	3	have with fruit or salad
Tesco Cumberland Fish Bake	around 240 g (¼ pack)	3	accompany with lots of veg
Tortellini, Cheese	12 tortellini	3	remember to add any GiPs from sauces
Vine Leaves, Stuffed with Rice	8 medium vine leaves	3	
Beans, Mung, Green, Gram, Cooked Dahl	1 teacupful	3.5	use as little oil as possible if cooking from scratch
Lamb/Beef Hot Pot with Potatoes, chilled/frozen	ready meal portion	3.5	look out for supermarket healthier versions

For simplicity, a teacupful is just a standard teacup you may have at home
For ease of reference, 1 serving spoon = 3 tablespoons

Food	Portion Size	Total GiPs	Special Comments
Pizza, cheese and tomato, deep pan	2 slices from medium (9" diameter) or 1 slice of large (12" diameter)	3.5	GI of other pizza toppings not available – if choosing meat toppings, opt for lower-fat types
Pizza, cheese and tomato, thin base	2 slices from medium (9" diameter) or 1 slice of large (12" diameter)	3.5	GI of other pizza toppings not available – if choosing meat toppings, avoid extra cheese
Pizza, vegetarian	2 slices from medium (9" diameter) or 1 slice of large (12" diameter)	3.5	choose less cheese and more veggies
Sainsbury's Be Good to Yourself Chicken Tikka Masala & Rice	per pack	3.5	have with salad
Tesco Chicken Szechuan	350 g	3.5	count GiPs from accompaniments
Tesco Healthy Living Lasagne	340 g	3.5	
Chicken nuggets, take-away	6 nuggets	4	high in salt
Cornish pasty	1 pasty	4	pastry is high in fat, go easy
Macaroni cheese	2 serving spoons	4	tomato-based sauces tend to be lower in calories and richer in antioxidants
Sainsbury's Be Good to Yourself Tuna and Cucumber Sandwich	per pack	4	have with salad and/or fruit
Tesco Healthy Living Chicken Chow Mein	450 g	4	
Tesco Italiano tomato and mozzarella pasta bake	340 g	4	have with salad and/or fruit
Chicken, stir-fried with rice and vegetables, frozen	ready meal portion	4.5	choose supermarket healthier version
Steak and kidney/Beef pie, individual, chilled/frozen, baked	1 pie	4.5	
Tesco Chicken Fajitas	275 g (½ pack)	4.5	keep to portion size
Tesco Finest Lasagne	300 g (½ pack)	4.5	
Tesco Spinach & Ricotta Cannelloni	400 g (½ pack)	5	try recipe, 4 GiPs

For simplicity, a teacupful is just a standard teacup you may have at home
For ease of reference, 1 serving spoon = 3 tablespoons

| Food | Portion Size | Total GiPs | Special Comments |

ALPHABETICAL GiP TABLE

BEANS AND LENTILS *all beans and lentils are carbohydrates and count once a day as one of your five daily fruit and veg. These are also protein foods and if you choose them as your protein, then choose another carb.*

BREAKFAST CEREALS *you will find all breakfast cereals under C for cereal. Also see low combo breakfasts (page 308)*

EGGS *max 5-6 per week, try omega-3 types. Have less if medically advised to do so*

FATS AND OILS *opt for monounsaturated ones*

FATTY AND SUGARY FOODS *keep to a minimum*

FISH *choose fish twice a week, one being oily fish, which is rich in omega-3 fats*

FRUIT *have five fruit and veg a day: they're rich in antioxidants*

FRUITS, DESSERTS, SNACKS, DRINKS *fruit gets the gold star*

MEAL CARBS *choose one at each meal*

NUTS *use nuts in cooking to provide protein*

PASTA *most pasta is very low GI. Use 50 g raw per portion*

PROTEIN *choose 2–3 portions a day*

RICE AND GRAINS *keep rice grains whole rather than soft and mushy. Use 45 g raw per serving*

SNACKS *nuts in shells take longer to eat, so you may end up having less*

STARCHY VEGETABLES *these are part of meal carbs since they are high in starch. Other vegetables are not – you can find these under Vegetables*

VEGETABLES *packed with GiP-free choices*

A

Food	Portion Size	Total GiPs	Special Comments
Ackee, canned, drained	½ can	2	
Alfalfa sprouts	as desired	0	
Almonds	10–12 almonds	3	high in fat but low in GI and saturates, choose nuts once a day strictly in these amounts
Apples	1 apple	0.5	the whole fruit has all the fibre, choose it over fruit juice
Apricots, dried	4 apricots	2	good source of fibre and beta-carotene
Apricots, fresh	4 apricots	2.5	

For simplicity, a teacupful is just a standard teacup you may have at home
For ease of reference, 1 serving spoon = 3 tablespoons

Food	Portion Size	Total GiPs	Special Comments
Artichoke, globe	as desired	0	
Artificial sweeteners		0	if you have a lot, vary the types
Asparagus	as desired	0	
Asparagus, canned, drained	as desired	0	
Aubergines, grilled	as desired	0	
Avocado	1 small	2	

B

Babybel cheese, mini, light	1 individual portion	2.5	
Bacon rashers, back, grilled	3 rashers	3	GI of turkey rashers is not available, but they are a lower-fat choice
Bacon rashers, middle, grilled	3 rashers	3.5	
Bacon, gammon joint, lean only, cooked	140 g steak	2	cooked weight, high in salt, limit amounts
Bagels, plain	1 bagel	6	a low-GiP carb filling (like sweetcorn) helps to reduce the GI of the meal
Baked beans, canned in tomato sauce	1 small can	2	
Baked Beans, Tesco Healthy Living	220 g can	1	
Bamboo shoots, canned, drained	as desired	0	
Banana bread	1 slice	4.5	
Bananas	1 small banana	2	great source of potassium
Barley, pearl, cooked	1 teacupful	1.5	throw some into soups and stews
Beef sausages, grilled	2 sausages	3	GI of lower-fat sausages is not available, but they are a better choice
Beef sirloin joint, roasted lean	3 slices	2	
Beef stew, made with lean beef	2 serving spoons	1.5	limit or avoid fat in cooking
Beef, mince, stewed	2 serving spoons	2.5	choose lean beef

For simplicity, a teacupful is just a standard teacup you may have at home
For ease of reference, 1 serving spoon = 3 tablespoons

Food	Portion Size	Total GiPs	Special Comments
Beef, rump steak, lean, grilled	140 g steak	2	cooked weight
Beef, topside, roasted well-done, lean	3 slices	2.5	
Beefburgers, chilled/frozen, grilled	2 beefburgers	3.5	
Beetroot, cooked	4 slices	2.5	
Beetroot, pickled, drained	4 slices	2	
Black gram, urad gram, dried, cooked	1 teacupful	2	
Blackeye beans, dried, cooked	1 teacupful	1.5	GI of some canned beans is not available
Blue Stilton cheese	matchbox-size piece (25 g)	4.5	
Bread, baguette	1 individual	9	a great food but a very high GI. Eat always with a low-GiP carb (like salad)
Bread, barley	2 slices	3	
Bread, barley and sunflower	2 slices	4.5	
Bread, Burgen soya and linseed	2 slices	2.5	grains and seeds tend to lower the GI
Bread, granary	2 slices	3.5	
Bread, hamburger buns	1 bun	5	
Bread, Hovis	2 slices	5.5	
Bread, Irwin's Low GI White	2 slices	2.5	contains added ingredients which lower the GI; only available in Northern Ireland at time of going to press
Bread, mixed grain	2 slices	3.5	wholegrains are richer in B vitamins than refined grains
Bread, pitta	1 pitta	5	wholemeal ones are higher in fibre
Bread, pitta, Sainsbury's mini	1 mini pitta	2.5	
Bread, pitta, Sainsbury's wholemeal	1 pitta	4.5	
Bread, Pumpernickel	2 slices	3.5	
Bread, rye	2 slices	4.5	
Bread, Warburtons All In One bread	2 slices	3.5	contains added ingredients which lower the GI

For simplicity, a teacupful is just a standard teacup you may have at home
For ease of reference, 1 serving spoon = 3 tablespoons

Food	Portion Size	Total GIPs	Special Comments
Bread, Warburtons All In One Rolls	1 roll	2	
Bread, Warburtons All In One Riddlers	1 roll	3.5	
Bread, white	2 slices	5.5	
Bread, white, with added fibre	2 slices	4.5	
Bread, wholemeal	2 slices	5.5	opt for stoneground as it is more coarse and thus has a lower GI
Breadfruit, boiled	2 slices	3.5	
Breadfruit, canned, drained	2 slices	3	
Breakfast cereals – see Cereal			
Brie cheese	matchbox-size piece (25 g)	3.5	
Bright Bar Energise	1 bar (35 g)	3.5	
Bright Bar Inside	1 bar (35 g)	3.5	
Broad beans, boiled	2 tbsp	3.5	
Broad beans, canned	½ large can	4	great with red onion
Broad beans, dried, cooked	1 teacupful	3.5	
Broad beans, frozen, cooked	1 teacupful	4	
Broccoli, green, frozen, steamed	as desired	0	
Broccoli, green, raw	as desired	0	contains iron
Broccoli, green, steamed	as desired	0	
Broccoli, purple sprouting, steamed	as desired	0	
Brussels sprouts, frozen, steamed	12 sprouts	0	
Brussels sprouts, steamed	12 sprouts	0	
Bulgur, cooked	1 teacupful (50 g raw)	2	one of the lowest-GI grains, see recipes
Butter	scraping	1	
Butter beans, dried, boiled	½ can	1.5	
Butter beans, dried, cooked	1 teacupful	1.5	

C

Food	Portion Size	Total GIPs	Special Comments
Cabbage, spring, steamed	as desired	0	
Cabbage, winter, steamed	as desired	0	
Cabbage, Chinese, raw	as desired	0	
Cabbage, frozen, steamed	as desired	0	

For simplicity, a teacupful is just a standard teacup you may have at home
For ease of reference, 1 serving spoon = 3 tablespoons

Food	Portion Size	Total GiPs	Special Comments
Cabbage, raw	as desired	0	raw is a good source of vitamin C
Cabbage, red, steamed	as desired	0	
Cabbage, Savoy, steamed	as desired	0	
Cabbage, summer, steamed	as desired	0	
Cabbage, white, steamed	as desired	0	
Camembert cheese	matchbox-size piece (25 g)	3	lower in fat than Brie
Cannellini beans, Tesco	½ can (150 g)	2.5	
Carrot, average raw	1 large carrot	0.5	
Carrots, fresh, steamed	2 tbsp	0.5	
Cashew nuts	15 cashews	3.5	high in fat but low in GI, choose nuts once a day strictly in these amounts
Cassava, baked	size of a medium potato	3	available frozen in some supermarkets; frozen ones may have added fat, check labels
Cassava, boiled	size of a medium potato	2.5	you can buy cassava frozen in Asian shops
Cassava, steamed	size of a medium potato	2.5	
Cauliflower, frozen, steamed	as desired	0	
Cauliflower, raw	as desired	0	
Cauliflower, steamed	as desired	0	
Crackers, wholemeal	2 crackers	3	
Celeriac, raw	as desired	0	
Celeriac, steamed	as desired	0	
Celery, raw	as desired	0	source of potassium
Celery, steamed	as desired	0	
Cereal chewy bar – dried fruit	45–50 g bar	4.5	
Cereal crunchy bar – dried fruit	45–50 g bar	4.5	
Cereal, All Bran and semi-skimmed milk	5 tbsp + 200 ml (⅓ pint)	2	try it with sliced banana
Cereal, Bran Flakes and semi-skimmed milk	4 tbsp + 200 ml (⅓ pint)	4	

For simplicity, a teacupful is just a standard teacup you may have at home
For ease of reference, 1 serving spoon = 3 tablespoons

Food	Portion Size	Total GiPs	Special Comments
Cereal, cornflakes and semi-skimmed milk	5 tbsp+ 200 ml (⅓ pint)	4.5	
Cereal, Fruit & Fibre Breakfast, Tesco and semi-skimmed milk	4 tbsp (40 g) + 200 ml (⅓ pint)	4.5	
Cereal, Grapenuts and semi-skimmed milk	5 tbsp + 200 ml (⅓ pint)	4.5	
Cereal, Hi Fibre Bran Breakfast, Tesco and semi-skimmed milk	30 g + 200 ml (⅓ pint)	2	
Cereal, instant hot oats made with semi-skimmed milk	follow pack instructions using 200 ml (⅓ pint) milk	4.5	a sachet at work could be a convenient breakfast
Cereal, muesli and semi-skimmed milk	4 tbsp (40 g) + 200 ml (⅓ pint)	4	
Cereal, muesli, reduced sugar and semi-skimmed milk	4 tbsp (40 g) + 200 ml (⅓ pint)	4	
Cereal, muesli, Swiss style and semi-skimmed milk	4 tbsp (40 g) + 200 ml (⅓ pint)	4	
Cereal, muesli, Tesco Value and semi-skimmed milk	40 g + 200 ml (⅓ pint)	3.5	about 4 tbsp
Cereal, Nutrigrain and semi-skimmed milk	5 tbsp + 200 ml (⅓ pint)	4.5	
Cereal, oats, Sainsbury's Taste the Difference Scottish jumbo oats and semi-skimmed milk	40 g + 150 ml	3.5	GI-tested on this amount, but use 30 g if you prefer it less thick
Cereal, porridge, made with milk and water	6 tbsp of made-up porridge using 100 ml milk and water as required	3.5	you could try skimmed milk, 200 ml (⅓ pint), instead. Use a little sweetener, honey or fructose if you like, add the GiPs
Cereal, porridge, made with water	8 tbsp of made-up porridge as pack instructions	3	quick microwaveable breakfast. Try Speedy Porridge with Grated Apple, see recipes
Cereal, Puffed Wheat and semi-skimmed milk	5 tbsp + 200 ml (⅓ pint)	4	a good bowl of fibre
Cereal, Raisin Splitz and semi-skimmed milk	4 tbsp + 200 ml (⅓ pint)	4.5	
Cereal, Rice Krispies and semi-skimmed milk	7 tbsp + 200 ml (⅓ pint)	5.5	

For simplicity, a teacupful is just a standard teacup you may have at home
For ease of reference, 1 serving spoon = 3 tablespoons

Food	Portion Size	Total GiPs	Special Comments
Cereal, Sainsbury's Precise and semi-skimmed milk	40 g + 150 ml	4.5	GI-tested on this amount of cereal and milk
Cereal, Shredded Wheat and semi-skimmed milk	2 biscuits + 200 ml (⅓ pint)	4.5	
Cereal, Special K and semi-skimmed milk	5 tbsp + 200 ml (⅓ pint)	4	most cereals are enriched with vitamins
Cereal, Sultana Bran and semi-skimmed milk	4 tbsp + 200 ml (⅓ pint)	4.5	
Cereal, Weetabix and semi-skimmed milk	2 biscuits + 200 ml (⅓ pint)	4.5	cereal for breakfast means you get calcium from milk
Chapatis, made with fat	2 small chapatis	5.5	
Chapatis, made without fat	2 small chapatis	4.5	use coarse wholemeal flour
Chard, Swiss, raw	as desired	0	
Chard, Swiss, steamed	as desired	0	
Cheddar cheese	matchbox-size piece (25 g)	4.5	grated goes further, use 3 tbsp
Cheddar cheese, half-fat	matchbox-size piece (25 g)	3	
Cherries	12 cherries	0.5	
Cheshire cheese	matchbox-size piece (25 g)	4	
Chick peas, canned	½ large can	2	great spiced up as a snack – add chilli sauce and lemon
Chick peas, split, dried, cooked	1 teacupful	2.5	
Chick peas, whole, dried, cooked	1 teacupful	1.5	
Chicken Chow Mein, Tesco Healthy Living	450 g	4	
Chicken Fajitas, Tesco	275 g (½ pack)	4.5	keep to portion size
Chicken nuggets, frozen	6 nuggets	4	bake your own with chicken breast, spices and olive oil spray
Chicken nuggets, take-away	6 nuggets	4	
Chicken Szechuan, Tesco	350 g	3.5	count GiPs from accompaniments

For simplicity, a teacupful is just a standard teacup you may have at home
For ease of reference, 1 serving spoon = 3 tablespoons

Food	Portion Size	Total GiPs	Special Comments
Chicken Tikka Masala & Rice, Sainsbury's Be Good to Yourself	per pack	3.5	have with salad
Chicken, breast chunks or strips	2 serving spoons	2	
Chicken, breast, skinless, roasted	1 medium	2	
Chicken, drumstick, skinless, roasted	2 drumsticks	2	higher in fat than chicken breast
Chicken, leg, skinless, roasted	1 medium	2	
Chicken, roasted	3 slices	2	try the Citrus Roast Chicken recipe
Chicken, stir-fried with rice and vegetables, frozen	ready meal portion	4.5	
Chicken, thigh, skinless, roasted	1 medium	2	
Chicken, wing, skinless, roasted	4 wings	2	
Chicory, raw	as desired	0	
Chicory, steamed	as desired	0	
Chilli beans, canned	½ large can	1	
Chilli sauce	as desired	0	
Chips, French fries, fast food outlet	2 serving spoons	6	
Chips, straight cut, frozen, oven baked	2 serving spoons	5	choose 5% fat varieties
Chocolate, milk	1 square piece	1.5	
Chocolate, milk	1 treat-size bar (15 g)	2	
Chocolate, white	1 treat-size bar (13 g)	2	
Chocolate-covered peanuts (e.g. M&M)	1 small pack (47 g)	5	
Cockles	6 cockles	1	
Cod, baked	1 fillet	1	try the Lemony Cod recipe
Cod, grilled	1 fillet	1	
Coffee, no sugar	as desired	0	use milk from allowance
Corn chips	small packet (30 g)	6	try the 3-GiP Crispy Tortilla Chips recipe
Corned beef, canned	2 slices	2.5	watch the salt!
Cornish pasty	1 pasty	4	pastry is high in fat, go easy

For simplicity, a teacupful is just a standard teacup you may have at home
For ease of reference, 1 serving spoon = 3 tablespoons

Food	Portion Size	Total GiPs	Special Comments
Cottage cheese, plain	small tub	1.5	
Cottage cheese, plain, reduced fat	small tub	1	
Courgette, cooked in spray oil	as desired	0	use 5 sprays of oil. See the recipe for Chargrilled Courgette Ribbons
Courgette, raw	as desired	0	
Courgette, sautéed	1 courgette	1	or use spray oil and count as 0
Courgette, steamed	as desired	0	
Couscous, cooked	1 teacupful	3.5	a nice change from rice. Try the Nutty Couscous recipe
Crab	2 tbsp crab meat	1.5	
Cream cheese – see Soft cheese			
Cream crackers	2 crackers	3	
Crème fraîche, half fat	50 ml	2	watch portion size
Crispbread, rye	2 crispbread	3	
Crisps, potato	small packet (25 g)	6.5	
Croissants	1 croissant	6	
Crumpets	1 crumpet	4	
Cucumber, raw	as desired	0	
Cumberland Fish Bake, Tesco	around 240 g (¼ pack)	3	accompany with lots of veg
Curly kale, steamed	as desired	0	
Currant bread (fruit loaf)	2 slices	4	no butter please!
Currant bun	1 bun	4	
Custard apple	1 custard apple	2	
Custard made with semi-skimmed milk	small yoghurt-pot size	1	

D

Food	Portion Size	Total GiPs	Special Comments
Danish pastries	Small pastry	5.5	pastry is often rich in trans fats
Dates, dried	4 dates	2	
Dhokra, Indian	4 pieces	2	

For simplicity, a teacupful is just a standard teacup you may have at home
For ease of reference, 1 serving spoon = 3 tablespoons

Food	Portion Size	Total GiPs	Special Comments
Diet soft drinks	as desired	0	you could go for decaff versions
Digestive biscuits, plain	1 biscuit	3.5	reduced-fat versions are available
Doughnuts, ring	1 doughnut	7.5	
Dressing, fat-free	limit to about 2 tbsp	0	
Duck, roasted	3 slices	2	avoid the skin

E

Food	Portion Size	Total GiPs	Special Comments
Edam cheese	matchbox-size piece (25 g)	2.5	
Eggs, boiled	2 eggs	1.5	
Eggs, fried	1 egg	1.5	or use 10 sprays of oil and count as boiled
Eggs, poached	2 eggs	1.5	
Eggs, scrambled, with milk and 1 tsp oil	2 eggs	3	
Emmental cheese	matchbox-size piece (25 g)	4	
Endive, raw	as desired	0	

F

Food	Portion Size	Total GiPs	Special Comments
Fennel, raw	as desired	0	
Fennel, steamed	as desired	0	
Feta cheese	matchbox-size piece (25 g)	2.5	
Figs, dried	2 figs	3	
Fish fingers, cod, grilled	4 fingers	2	or freeze your own cod strips, try the Lemony Cod Strips recipe
Flageolet beans, Tesco	½ can (150 g)	2.5	throw beans into soups and stews
French fries – see Chips			
Fromage frais, virtually fat free	150 ml pot	1.5	
Fructose	2 tsp	1	

For simplicity, a teacupful is just a standard teacup you may have at home
For ease of reference, 1 serving spoon = 3 tablespoons

Food	Portion Size	Total GiPs	Special Comments
Fruit cocktail, canned in juice	½ large can	1	
Fruit loaf – see Currant bread			

G

Gherkins, pickled, drained	as desired	0	
Glucose – liquid	2 tsp	9.5	goes straight into the bloodstream!
Glucose drink, sparkling	1 glass (150 ml)	7	
GoLower Nut Bar – Chocolate	34 g	3	no extra nuts on this day
GoLower Nut Bar – Coconut	34 g	3	no extra nuts on this day
GoLower Nut Bar – Raspberry	34 g	3	no extra nuts on this day
Gourd, kantola, canned, drained	as desired	0	
Gourd, karela, canned, drained	as desired	0	
Gourd, tinda, canned, drained	as desired	0	
Grapefruit	1 grapefruit	0	rich in potassium which helps to regulate blood pressure
Grapes	15 grapes	2	
Gravy, instant	2 serving spoons	0.5	can be high in salt, but lower in fat than using meat juices

H

Haddock, smoked	1 fillet	1.5	smoked foods are higher in salt, so limit amounts
Haddock, steamed or grilled	1 fillet	1	
Halibut, steamed or grilled	1 fillet	1.5	
Ham	2 slices	1.5	
Haricot beans, dried, cooked	1 teacupful	1	
Haricot beans, dried, steamed	1 teacupful	1	
Herbs, fresh or dried		0	
Herring, grilled	2 fillets	2	a source of healthy omega-3 fats
Honey	1 tsp	1	
Hummus, half-fat	¼ pot, 2 tbsp	2	

For simplicity, a teacupful is just a standard teacup you may have at home
For ease of reference, 1 serving spoon = 3 tablespoons

Food	Portion Size	Total GiPs	Special Comments
I			
Ice cream, dairy, vanilla	1 scoop	2	or freeze diet yoghurt for 4 hours, 1 GiP
Ice cream, reduced-calorie	1 scoop	1.5	add some lemon zest for zing
innocent kids Oranges, Mangoes and Pineapples	180 ml carton	1.5	keep to portion size
innocent Mangoes and Passionfruit	150 ml (small glass)	2	pour this amount from a litre pack
innocent Strawberries and Bananas	150 ml (small glass)	2	pour this amount from a litre pack
J			
Jacob Essentials – Wholewheat crackers with sesame seeds & rosemary	2 triangles	2	or have one for 1 GiP
Jam	1 tsp	1	
Jam, reduced sugar	1 tsp	0.5	
Jelly, sugar-free	as desired	0	
Jellybeans	6 jelly beans	4	
Juice, apple unsweetened	1 glass (150 ml)	1	keep to portion size, cloudy has a slightly lower GI
Juice, cranberry	1 glass (150 ml)	3	diet versions are lower in calories, but GI value is not available
Juice, grapefruit, unsweetened	1 glass (150 ml)	1.5	
Juice, orange, unsweetened	1 glass (150 ml)	1.5	
Juice, pineapple, unsweetened	1 glass (150 ml)	1.5	
Juice, tomato	1 glass (150 ml)	0	add some Worcester sauce for a bit of zing!
K			
Kidney, lamb, sautéed	2 kidneys	2	
Kidney, ox, stewed	3 tbsp	1.5	
Kipper, baked	2 fillets	2.5	a source of healthy omega-3 fats, but high in salt

For simplicity, a teacupful is just a standard teacup you may have at home
For ease of reference, 1 serving spoon = 3 tablespoons

Food	Portion Size	Total GiPs	Special Comments
Kiwi fruit	1 kiwi	0.5	abundant in vitamin C
Kohl rabi, raw	as desired	0	
Kohl rabi, steamed	as desired	0	

L

Food	Portion Size	Total GiPs	Special Comments
Lamb, breast, roasted, lean	3 slices	3	
Lamb, leg joint, roasted, lean	3 slices	2.5	
Lamb, loin chops, grilled, lean	2 chops	1.5	try the Minty Lamb Chops recipe
Lamb, scrag and neck, lean only, stewed	2 serving spoons	1.5	limit or avoid fat in cooking
Lamb, shoulder joint, roasted, lean	3 slices	2.5	
Lamb/Beef Hot Pot with Potatoes, chilled/frozen	ready meal portion	3.5	look out for supermarket healthier versions
Lasagne, Tesco Finest	300 g (½ pack)	4.5	
Lasagne, Tesco Healthy Living	340 g	3.5	
Leeks, steamed	as desired	0	
Lemon sole, steamed or grilled	1 fillet	1	
Lentils, green, Tesco	½ can (150 g)	1	try the dahl recipes
Lentils, red, split, dried, cooked	1 teacupful	1	
Lettuce, butterhead, raw	as desired	0	
Lettuce, Cos, raw	as desired	0	
Lettuce, Iceberg, raw	as desired	0	
Lettuce, mixed leaves	as desired	0	
Lettuce, Webbs, raw	as desired	0	
Liver sausage	1 slice	2.5	all sausages tend to be high in salt and very processed
Liver, lamb, sautéed	2 slices	2.5	rich in iron, great for the immune system
Liver, ox, stewed	3 tbsp	2	rich in iron and vitamin B^{12}
Lobster	2 tbsp	1.5	flavour with lemon juice
Lotus tubers, canned	as desired	0	

For simplicity, a teacupful is just a standard teacup you may have at home
For ease of reference, 1 serving spoon = 3 tablespoons

Food	Portion Size	Total GiPs	Special Comments

M

Food	Portion Size	Total GiPs	Special Comments
Mackerel, canned in brine, drained	1 small can	2.5	a source of healthy omega-3 fats
Mangoes	1 small mango	2	try the Mango Smoothie recipe
Marmalade, reduced sugar	1 tsp	0.5	
Marrow, parwal, canned, drained	as desired	0	
Marrow, steamed	as desired	0	filling and low in calories
Mars® bar	1 fun-size (19 g)	3	
Matoki, boiled	1 matoki	4	available from Asian/West Indian food stores
Mayonnaise, reduced calorie	1 tbsp	3	or count 1 tsp as 1 GiP
Melba toast, plain	2 toasts	7	
Melon, cantaloupe	½ melon	2	
Melon, watermelon	1 slice	3.5	
Milk, flavoured, Chocolate Nesquik made with semi-skimmed milk	200 ml (⅓ pint)	2	
Milk, flavoured, chocolate, reduced fat	200 ml (⅓ pint)	1	
Milk, flavoured, Strawberry Nesquik made with semi-skimmed milk	200 ml (⅓ pint)	1	GI has been analysed on this brand, but you can choose any brand if you like
Milk, semi-skimmed	200 ml (⅓ pint)	0.5	
Milk, skimmed	200 ml (⅓ pint)	0.5	
Mini-wheats, Sainsbury's wholegrain and semi-skimmed milk	40 g + 150 ml	3.5	GI-tested on this amount of cereal and milk
Mixed Beans Italienne, Tesco	½ can (150 g)	1	
Mooli – see Radish, white			
Mousse, reduced-fat	1 small pot	1.5	
Mozzarella cheese	matchbox-size piece (25 g)	3	
Muffins, American style, chocolate chip	1 muffin	5	choosing a smaller one means fewer calories
Muffins, blueberry	1 muffin	5	

For simplicity, a teacupful is just a standard teacup you may have at home
For ease of reference, 1 serving spoon = 3 tablespoons

Food	Portion Size	Total GiPs	Special Comments
Muffins, oat bran	1 muffin	5	
Mung beans, green, gram, cooked dahl	1 teacupful	3.5	use as little oil as possible if cooking from scratch
Mung beans, whole, dried, cooked	1 teacupful	2	
Mushroom burger, Tesco	87.5 g (½ pack)	2.5	grill to keep the fat down
Mushrooms, raw	as desired	0	
Mushrooms, canned, drained	as desired	0	
Mushrooms, common, stir-fried	2 tbsp	2	or use spray oil, 0 GiPs
Mushrooms, oyster, raw	as desired	0	
Mushrooms, steamed	as desired	0	
Mushrooms, straw, canned, drained	as desired	0	
Mussels	6 mussels	1.5	
Mustard and cress, raw	as desired	0	
Mustard leaves, steamed	as desired	0	
Mustard, any type		0	

N

Food	Portion Size	Total GiPs	Special Comments
New potatoes, boiled	4 new potatoes	3	keep skins on
New potatoes, canned, drained	4 new potatoes	3	
Noodles, instant, cooked	50 g dried/ 115 g cooked	2	
Noodles, rice, cooked	5 tbsp (50 g dried)	3	
Nougat	4 sweets	4	

O

Food	Portion Size	Total GiPs	Special Comments
Oat cakes	1 oat cake	1	oats are low GI
Oil, olive oil	1 tsp	1.5	monounsaturated
Oil, rapeseed oil	1 tsp	1.5	monounsaturated. Also sometimes sold as vegetable oil – check label
Oil, spray oil	see special comments	0	up to 10 sprays per dish, strict portion limit
Oil, sunflower oil	1 tsp	2	if cooking for 4, use 4 tsp and then count your portion as 2 GiPs

For simplicity, a teacupful is just a standard teacup you may have at home
For ease of reference, 1 serving spoon = 3 tablespoons

Food	Portion Size	Total GiPs	Special Comments
Oil, vegetable oil, mixed	1 tsp	2	
Okra, canned, drained	as desired	0	
Okra, steamed	as desired	0	
Old potatoes, baked	1 medium potato	7	
Old potatoes, boiled	3 egg-size potatoes	3	cold cooked potatoes have a lower GI!
Olives	10 olives	0.5	olives with stones take longer to eat so you might eat less
Omelette, plain, made with 1 tsp oil	2 eggs	3	
Onions, cooked	as desired	0	
Onions, pickled, cocktail/silverskin, drained	as desired	0	
Oranges	1 large orange	1.5	the GI of satsumas is not available, but you can choose 2–3 satsumas instead of an orange and count the GiPs as 1.5
Oxtail, stewed	2 serving spoons	2.5	
Oysters	1 dozen oysters	1	shellfish are a good source of zinc, great for immune function

P

Food	Portion Size	Total GiPs	Special Comments
Pak Choi	as desired	0	great in soups (see Hot and Sour Soup recipe)
Parsnip, boiled	2 tbsp	7	serve with low-GiP veggies
Parsnip, roast	2 tbsp	7.5	
Parsnip, steamed	2 tbsp	7	a great veg, but high in GI
Pasta, egg tagliatelle	5 tbsp (50 g dried)	3	
Pasta, fettuccine, egg, cooked	5 tbsp (50 g dried)	1.5	try the Fettuccine recipe
Pasta, Fusilli Twists, Tesco	5 tbsp (50 g dried)	3	
Pasta, linguini, thick, cooked	50 g dried/ 115 g cooked	2.5	make a low-fat tomato and basil sauce (page 263)

For simplicity, a teacupful is just a standard teacup you may have at home
For ease of reference, 1 serving spoon = 3 tablespoons

Food	Portion Size	Total GiPs	Special Comments
Pasta, linguini, thin, cooked	50 g dried/ 115 g cooked	2.5	
Pasta, macaroni cheese	2 serving spoons	4	tomato-based sauces tend to be lower in calories and richer in antioxidants
Pasta, macaroni, cooked	5 tbsp (50 g dried)	2	
Pasta, Italiano tomato and mozzarella pasta bake, Tesco	340 g	4	have with salad and/or fruit
Pasta, plain, cooked	5 tbsp (50 g dried)	3	team pasta up with lower-fat tomato-based sauce, compare labels
Pasta, Ravioli, meat	12 ravioli	1.5	
Pasta, spaghetti, white, cooked	50 g dried/ 115 g cooked	1.5	cook till *al dente* (firm to the bite)
Pasta, spaghetti, wholemeal, cooked	50 g dried/ 115 g cooked	1.5	try the Garlic Spaghetti recipe
Pasta, Spinach & Ricotta Cannelloni, Tesco	400 g	5	
Pasta, tortellini, cheese	12 tortellini	3	remember to add any GiPs from sauces
Paw-paw	½ small	2.5	
Peaches	1 peach	1.5	
Peaches, canned in juice	6 slices	0.5	
Peanuts, dry roasted	pub pack (25 g) or half 50 g pack	3	high in fat but low in saturates and GI, choose nuts once a day strictly in these amounts
Peanuts, in shells	15 shells	3	shells help you limit intake and nuts are unsalted
Peanuts, roasted and salted	pub pack (25 g) or half 50 g pack	3	high in fat but low in saturates and GI, choose nuts once a day strictly in these amounts
Pears	1 pear	0.5	
Pears, canned in juice	2 pear halves	1.5	
Peas, fresh, steamed	3 tbsp	2	
Peas, frozen, steamed	3 tbsp	2	source of protein

For simplicity, a teacupful is just a standard teacup you may have at home
For ease of reference, 1 serving spoon = 3 tablespoons

Food	Portion Size	Total GIPs	Special Comments
Pecan nuts	12 halves	3	choose nuts once a day stictly in these amounts
Pepper, any type	as desired	0	
Peppers, capsicum, steamed	as desired	0	
Peppers, raw	as desired	0	rich in vitamin C
Pigeon peas, whole, dried, cooked	1 teacupful	1.5	
Pineapple	1 slice	2.5	
Pinto beans, dried, cooked	1 teacupful	1.5	a low-GI wonder food
Pitta bread – see Bread			
Pizza, cheese and tomato, deep pan	2 slices from medium (9" diameter) or 1 slice of large (12" diameter)	3.5	GI of other pizza toppings not available – if choosing meat toppings, opt for lower-fat types
Pizza, cheese and tomato, thin base	2 slices from medium (9" diameter) or 1 slice of large (12" diameter)	3.5	GI of other pizza toppings not available – if choosing meat toppings – avoid extra cheese
Pizza, vegetarian	2 slices from medium (9" diameter) or 1 slice of large (12" diameter)	3.5	choose less cheese and more veggies
Plaice, steamed or grilled	1 fillet	1	
Plantain, boiled	1 plantain	1.5	choose unripe ones, available from West Indian food stores
Plantain, steamed	1 plantain	1.5	choose unripe variety
Plums	3 plums	0.5	
Pooris, Indian	2 pooris	7.5	deep fried, so have on occasion only
Popcorn, plain	5 tbsp	4	choose lower-fat varieties, or make your own
Pork leg joint, roasted	3 slices	2	
Pork sausages, grilled	2 sausages	3	
Pork, loin chops, grilled, lean	1 chop	2	
Porridge – see Cereal			

For simplicity, a teacupful is just a standard teacup you may have at home
For ease of reference, 1 serving spoon = 3 tablespoons

Food	Portion Size	Total GiPs	Special Comments
Potato, mashed, instant, made up with water	2 scoops	7	mashing carbs raises the GI; use the same GiP for homemade, add any GiPs from milk or butter
Prawns	1 small jar (125 g)	1	choose fat-free dressing
Pretzels	25 g portion	6	a low-fat snack but high in GI
Probiotic Original Drink , Tesco	100 ml	1	
Prunes, ready-to-eat	8 prunes	1.5	
Pumpkin, cooked	2 slices	3	
Q			
Quinoa	50 g raw/170 g cooked	2.5	use instead of rice
Quorn, pieces, as purchased	12 pieces	1	a great low-fat meat substitute, use the same GiP as two Quorn burgers
R			
Rabbit, stewed	2 serving spoons	1.5	
Raddiccio (salad leaves)	as desired	0	
Radish leaves, raw	as desired	0.5	
Radish, red, raw	as desired	0	
Radish, white/mooli, raw	as desired	0	
Raisins	1 tbsp	1	
Raspberries	1 teacupful	0	keep to portion size if you want to have them GiP-free
Red kidney beans, canned	½ large can	2	
Red kidney beans, dried, cooked	1 teacupful	1.5	you can use a combination of beans in smaller portions for the same GiPs
Rice cakes	2 cakes	7	calories per rice cake are low, but GI is high
Rice, brown, boiled	2 serving spoons	2.5	
Rice, white, Bangladeshi, boiled	2 serving spoons	1.5	available from Asian food stores

For simplicity, a teacupful is just a standard teacup you may have at home
For ease of reference, 1 serving spoon = 3 tablespoons

Food	Portion Size	Total GiPs	Special Comments
Rice, white, basmati, boiled	2 serving spoons	2.5	try the Aromatic Basmati rice recipe
Rice, white, easy cook, boiled	2 serving spoons	3.5	don't overcook
Rice, white, glutinous (sticky), boiled	2 serving spoons	7	
Rice, white, instant, boiled	2 serving spoons	3.5	
Rice, white, jasmin, boiled	2 serving spoons	7.5	
Rice, white, polished, boiled	2 serving spoons	3.5	
Rice, white, precooked, microwaved	2 serving spoons	2.5	
Rice, white, risotto, boiled	2 serving spoons	3.5	sticky rice has a higher GI so keep the grains separate
Rich tea	2 biscuits	2	
Ricotta cheese	small tub (150 g)	1.5	fantastic low-fat option
Runner beans, cooked	as desired	0	
Ryvita	2 crispbread	3	

S

Food	Portion Size	Total GiPs	Special Comments
Salmon, pink, canned in brine, drained	small can	2	a source of healthy omega-3 fats
Salmon, smoked	3 slices	1.5	a source of healthy omega-3 fats
Salmon, steamed or grilled	1 steak	2	try the salmon recipe (page 136)
Salt	cut down to taste	0	keep added salt to a minimum
Salt substitutes		0	about ⅔ less sodium than salt
Sandwich, Sainsbury's Be Good to Yourself Egg and Cress	per pack	3	have with fruit or salad
Sandwich, Sainsbury's Be Good to Yourself Tuna and Cucumber	per pack	4	have with salad and/or fruit
Sardines, canned in brine, drained	4 sardines	2	a source of healthy omega-3 fats
Sauerkraut	as desired	0	
Scallops, steamed	3 tbsp	1.5	
Scone, plain	1 scone	10	very high GI, hence high GiPs value

For simplicity, a teacupful is just a standard teacup you may have at home
For ease of reference, 1 serving spoon = 3 tablespoons

Food	Portion Size	Total GiPs	Special Comments
Scotch pancakes	2 pancakes	5	
Seakale, steamed	as desired	0	
Seaweed, nori, dried, raw	2 tbsp	1.5	contains the antioxidant selenium
Semolina, cooked dry	1 teacupful	4.5	
Sesame seeds	2 tsp	1	throw them into GiP-free salad for extra crunch
Shallots, raw	as desired	0	
Shortbread	2 fingers	7.5	
Shrimps	1 teacupful	1.5	
Shrimps, canned in brine, drained	1 small pot	1	
Snickers bar	1 fun size (19 g)	2	or cut a standard bar into 3
Soft cheese, medium-fat, (e.g. light version of cream cheese)	25 g	2	
Soup, lentil	1 soup bowl	2	wholesome and filling
Soup, minestrone, dried, as served	1 soup bowl	0	GI of only these packet soups is available, but you can try other flavours
Soup, noodle, instant	1 soup bowl	2	
Soup, tomato, cream of, canned	1 soup bowl	1	see GiP-free tomato soup recipe
Soup, tomato, dried, as served	1 soup bowl	0.5	
Soy sauce		0	try low-sodium types
Soya beans, dried, cooked	1 teacupful	1.5	
Soya, alternative to yoghurt, fruit	1 small pot	2	
Soya, non-dairy alternative to milk, unsweetened	200 ml (⅓ pint)	0.5	soya protein is rich in phytochemicals, shown to reduce blood cholesterol
Spices, fresh (e.g. garlic, ginger, chilli)	as desired	0	use crushed in jars for convenience
Spices, ground (e.g. paprika, chilli powder, curry powder)	as desired	0	try the Cajun-spiced Turkey recipe
Spices, whole (e.g. cumin seeds, coriander seeds, caraway seeds)	as desired	0	
Spinach, canned, drained	as desired	0	

For simplicity, a teacupful is just a standard teacup you may have at home
For ease of reference, 1 serving spoon = 3 tablespoons

Food	Portion Size	Total GiPs	Special Comments
Spinach, frozen, steamed	as desired	0	
Spinach, raw	as desired	0	cancer-protective
Spinach, steamed	as desired	0	
Sponge cake	small slice	6	watch portion size
Spread, half-fat, unsaturated	1 tsp	1	
Spread, half-fat, unsaturated	scraping	0.5	some are monounsaturated
Spread, low-fat	scraping	0.5	
Spread, low-fat	1 tsp	1	
Spread, very low-fat, unsaturated	1 tsp	0.5	
Spring greens, steamed	as desired	0	
Spring onions, bulbs and tops, raw	as desired	0	
Squash, sugar-free	as desired	0	
Steak and kidney/Beef pie, individual, chilled/frozen, baked	1 pie	4.5	
Stock cube		0	try low-sodium types
Strawberries	1 teacupful or 12	0	keep to portion size if you want to have them GiP-free
Sugar	2 tsp	2.5	
Sultanas	2 handfuls	3	
Sushi	6 mini	2.5	
Swede, steamed	2 tbsp	3	
Sweet potato, baked	1 small potato	3.5	
Sweet potato, boiled	1 small potato	3	a source of beta-carotene
Sweet potato, steamed	1 small potato	3	
Sweet potato, steamed or microwaved	1 small potato	3	
Sweetcorn, baby, canned, drained	as desired	0	throw into a stir-fry
Sweetcorn, baby, fresh and frozen, steamed	as desired	0	
Sweetcorn, kernels, canned, drained	3 tbsp	2.5	choose canned veg in unsalted, unsweetened water
Sweetcorn, kernels, fresh, cooked	3 tbsp	2.5	

For simplicity, a teacupful is just a standard teacup you may have at home
For ease of reference, 1 serving spoon = 3 tablespoons

Food	Portion Size	Total GiPs	Special Comments
Sweetcorn, on-the-cob, whole, steamed	1 sweetcorn	2	

T

Food	Portion Size	Total GiPs	Special Comments
Taco shells, baked	1 shell	7	
Tea, no sugar	as desired	0	use milk from allowance
Tofu, cooked	150 g	1	made from healthy soya beans but no fibre
Tomato purée		0	
Tomatoes, canned, with juice	as desired	0	rich in cancer-fighting lycopene
Tomatoes, cherry, raw	as desired	0	
Tomatoes, raw	as desired	0	make a sauce with spray oil, onion, garlic and herbs
Tongue, ox, stewed	2 slices	2.5	
Tortilla wrap	1 wrap	3	
Trout, steamed or grilled	1 fish	1.5	try the Thai-style Trout recipe
Tuna, canned in brine, drained	1 small can	1	half the calories of canned in oil
Turkey, roasted	2 slices	2	you get three times as much if you use wafer-thin turkey
Turnip, steamed	as desired	0	
Twix	1 mini Twix (21 g)	2.5	
Tzatziki	2 tbsp	1	opt for lower-fat versions if available

V

Food	Portion Size	Total GiPs	Special Comments
Veal, cutlet, sautéed	1 cutlet	2.5	use olive oil spray
Veal, fillet, roast	1 fillet	2.5	
Vegetables, Tesco Roasted Winter	200 g (½ pack)	2	
Vie Shot Apple/Carrot/Strawberry	100 ml	1	other flavours may have a different GI
Vie Shot Orange/Banana/Carrot	100 ml	2	

For simplicity, a teacupful is just a standard teacup you may have at home
For ease of reference, 1 serving spoon = 3 tablespoons

Food	Portion Size	Total GiPs	Special Comments
Vine leaves, preserved in brine	as desired	0	
Vine Leaves, stuffed with rice	8 medium vine leaves	3	
Vinegar (rice, balsamic, malt, wine)	as desired	0	

W

Waffles	1 waffle	6.5	
Walnuts	8 halves	3	throw them into salads, choose nuts once a day stictly in these amounts
Water biscuits	2 biscuits	7.5	calories per biscuit are low, but GI is high
Water, sparkling	as desired	0	
Water, still	as desired	0	
Water, sugar-free flavoured	as desired	0	check no added sugar
Watercress, raw	as desired	0	
Worcester sauce	as desired	0	

Y

Yam, baked	size of a medium potato	1.5	
Yam, boiled	size of a medium potato	1.5	
Yam, steamed	size of a medium potato	1.5	
Yoghurt, diet	1 small pot	1	
Yoghurt, drink	200 ml (⅓ pint)	1	choose reduced-calorie if available
Yoghurt, Greek, sheep's	150 ml	1	
Yoghurt, low-fat, Greek-style, natural	150 ml	1	
Yoghurt, low-fat, natural	small pot	1	
Yoghurt, Tesco Healthy Living Light Peach & Apricot	200g	0.5	
Yoghurt, Tesco Healthy Living Light Strawberry	200g	0.5	

For simplicity, a teacupful is just a standard teacup you may have at home
For ease of reference, 1 serving spoon = 3 tablespoons

10

PRACTICAL TOOLS

This is your very own practical tools section. It can be as tidy or as messy as you like. The aim is to use it as your private log that records all your achievements, activities, goals – and much more. We have inserted some blank pages, too, for your own personal notes.

Shopping List for the 'Easy-Menu'

If you've opted for the easy-menu choices, highlighted in bold, then here's your ready-made shopping list. We've made it even simpler for you by dividing your shopping spree into two days: one before you start your 10-day plan and one in the middle, around day 5 or 6, which falls on the weekend. This also helps you to preserve perishable items. You'll notice that the second shopping list is shorter as you will already have bought many of the items on the first trip.

❑ Before you begin, you will most likely have some of the items already (salt, pepper, etc), so do check your store-cupboard and fridge before you go out.

☐ You may also have some foods left over after the first trip, so you may not need to buy all the items on the second list.

☐ It is likely that some of the foods will last you longer than the 10 days, so you can keep to healthier low-GI eating after this time.

The list is arranged conveniently by supermarket aisles and similar foods appear together.

The amounts will generally serve one person, though obviously some of the pack sizes available will be larger than you require, especially in the case of herbs, sauces, dressings, packets of pasta, rice and so on. With other ingredients, we have sometimes indicated how much you will need for one person, so you can just adjust the quantity if you are serving more people.

Handy tips

There are plenty of handy shortcut tips in Chapter 3, *Getting Ready for Day 1*, but the one that you might find particularly useful is to freeze anything you can so it will last you for the rest of the 10 days and beyond (e.g. half a loaf of bread, tortilla wraps, bread rolls, leftover grated mozzarella cheese). There are also practical suggestions within the shopping list.

We hope to make this list available on our website (www.giplan.com) so you can take a copy and amend it if you wish.

Shopping trip one: days 1-5

Fresh fruit

Apples, 3
Banana, 1
Grapefruit, 1
Kiwi fruit, 1
Limes, 2
Pears, 2
Plums, 3
Satsumas, 2, or small pack
Strawberries, small punnet

Dried fruit, nuts and seeds

Prunes, ready-to-eat, small pack
Almonds, small pack
Sesame seeds, small pack

Fresh vegetables

Beansprouts, small pack
Button mushrooms, approx 325 g
French beans, 100 g needed (you can use more if you like)
Chillies, green, 4
Onions, 4 white, 1 red
Peppers, 3 red, 3 green, 1 yellow
Spring onions, 1 bunch
Tomatoes, approx 15
Aubergine, 1 (optional)

Courgette, 1 large

Asparagus tips, small pack

Pak Choi (Chinese leaves) or spinach leaves

Plus vegetables for salads and/or roasting. Buy your favourite combination of vegetables, for example, rocket leaves, cucumber, crispy lettuce, baby spinach leaves, watercress, celery, courgettes, radishes, cherry tomatoes, baby sweetcorn, baby gherkins, peppers, mushrooms, red onion, asparagus.

For home-made Marrow and Leek Soup, optional:

Marrow, 200 g

Leek, 1

Fresh herbs – basil, coriander, dill, mint, flat-leaf parsley (if you buy pots, remember to water them so they last longer)

Dressings

Fat-free dressing of your choice, small bottle

Fat-free Thai-style dressing, small bottle

Lemon or lime juice

Dairy chiller cabinet / chilled drinks

Low-fat spread, small tub (preferably unsaturated)

Cheese, Mozzarella, grated small pack OR Sainsbury's Be
    Good to Yourself Egg and Cress Sandwich (check use-by
    date: you need it for Wednesday, day 2)

Cheese, Ricotta, small tub

Milk, skimmed or semi-skimmed, around 1 to 2 litres, buy
    according to your usage

Tzatziki, small carton (optional, or use yoghurt already on list)

Yoghurt, diet, any flavour (if you buy more than four, this will
last you for the full 10 days, check use-by date)

Yoghurt, low-fat natural, 2 small pots or 1 large pot

Yoghurt, low-fat Greek style or Greek sheep's yoghurt, 150 ml
or a small pot

Tesco Probiotic Original Drink (low GI) – if you buy more
than one, you can opt for this choice on day 7 as shown,
use the rest after the initial 10 days, or share it!

Fruit juice, unsweetened, small carton

Tomato juice, if you like it

Vie Shot Apple/Carrot/Strawberry – if you buy more
than one, you can opt to have this on day 8 as shown,
use the rest after the initial 10 days (check use-by date),
or share it!

Fresh meat / fish / eggs

Chicken breast, 1 breast (you will need about half a breast:
you could cook it all and freeze the rest for another time,
or serve more than one person)

Eggs, pack of 6

Fresh trout fillet, 1

Minced beef, lean, 125 g (if you buy a larger pack, simply freeze
what you don't need; or cook for more than one serving
and freeze the leftovers)

Salmon, smoked, 3 slices

1 rasher grilled lean bacon (optional choice for cooked
breakfast; you can buy them singly at the meat counter)

Bread / bakery

(take out enough for the first few days and freeze the rest)

Bread, Burgen soya and linseed

Bread, granary, small loaf

Bread, multigrain, small loaf (or just use one of the above
loaves)

Tortilla wrap, wholemeal or white, standard pack

Canned vegetables / soups / fruit

Baby sweetcorn, I can

Kidney beans, I can (½ can needed for chilli con carne; you
could make twice the quantity, share it or freeze some
chilli for another day)

Soup, Minestrone, sachet (individual or a box so you can use
over a period of time, GiP-free)

Tomatoes, passata (sieved tomatoes), 250 ml needed, though
you can use more if pack size is bigger

Tomatoes, chopped, 2 cans

Bamboo shoots, I can

Water chestnuts, I can

Baked beans in tomato sauce, small can (optional choice for
vegetarian cooked breakfast)

Tesco Healthy Living baked beans, can, 220 g

Fruit cocktail, in juice, I can (½ standard can needed for one
person)

Cereals

Porridge oats, small pack; and/or any 4-GiP breakfast cereal of
your choice (see GiP tables)

Pasta, rice, grains and noodles

Pasta shells, small pack

Bulgur wheat, small pack

Noodles, thread egg noodles or instant noodles, small pack

Rice, basmati or brown, small pack

Dried beans and lentils

Red lentils, dried, small pack

Biscuits

(store enough for the 10 days in a separate airtight container; store the rest in another container which you will need after the initial 10 days)

Rich tea biscuits, small packet

Oatcakes, small packet

Jacob Essentials – Wholewheat crackers with sesame seeds
    & rosemary

Dried herbs, spices and flavourings

(these will last you for a long time and they are used often in the recipes)

Dried herbs: basil, parsley or herbs of your choice

Black pepper, coarse or cracked

Chinese five-spice powder

Red chilli powder, small pack

Mustard, coarse-grain (or regular, if preferred)

Reduced-fat tomato-based pasta sauce

Salt (try a salt substitute)

Soy sauce, small bottle (try reduced-salt versions)

Thai fish sauce

Vegetable stock, either vegetable bouillon OR stock cubes
   (try reduced-salt versions)

Worcester sauce

Curry powder, small pack

Cloves, small pack

Cinnamon sticks, small pack

Cumin seeds, small pack

Ground allspice, small pack

Ground coriander, small pack

Ground cinnamon, small pack

Ground garam masala, small pack

Ground turmeric, small pack

Ginger, crushed, 1 jar

Garlic, crushed, 1 jar

Spreads

Jam, reduced-sugar

Peanut butter, smooth or crunchy, preferably no added sugar

Miscellaneous

Artificial sweetener, if desired

Jelly, sugar-free, 2 pots

Milk chocolate bar, treat size (15 g)

Pickled onions, small jar (optional)

Spray oil, olive oil-based, 1 can

Frozen vegetables

If you prefer to buy frozen instead of fresh, check the vegetable section above and choose accordingly.

Drinks

Alcohol: wine (for 3 glasses over the 10 days) or beer (for 3 half-pint servings over the 10 days)
Coffee (as required)
Diet hot chocolate drink, sachets
Tea (any variety, as required)
Sugar-free drinks (as required)
Water (as required)

Shopping trip two: days 6–10

Check your store-cupboard/fridge for items that you may already have.

Fresh fruit

Apples, 1
Cherries, handful (optional, for cheesecake choice)
Grapes (small bunch – need 8–10)
Pears, 2
Satsumas, 2, or small pack (you may have some left over?)
Strawberries, small punnet

If you choose the banana and melon cocktail instead of cereal for Sunday breakfast:

Banana, under-ripe, 1

Cantaloupe melon, ½

Dried fruit, nuts and seeds

Apricots, dried, small pack

Peanuts in shells, roasted or raw, small pack (keep what you
don't need out of sight in an airtight container)

Fresh vegetables

(you may have some left over from your first shopping trip)

Cherry tomatoes, handful

Cucumber, 1 or a portion

Mixed salad leaves (e.g. rocket, iceberg, etc.)

Mushrooms, large flat, 2

Onion, 1

Peppers, 2

Spring onions, 2 or a bunch

Tomatoes, 7

Beef tomatoes, 2

Sweet potato (1 small) or new potatoes (4)

Plus vegetables for salads / roasting / GiP-free Veg Box. Buy
your favourite combination of vegetables. Here are some
examples: rocket leaves, cucumber, crispy lettuce, baby
spinach leaves, watercress, celery, courgettes, radishes,
cherry tomatoes, baby sweetcorn, baby gherkins, peppers,
mushrooms, red onion, asparagus, aubergine, mangetout

Plus unlimited vegetables for Sunday roast: e.g. cabbage,
spinach, broccoli, celeriac, courgettes, fennel, leeks, marrow,

peppers, spring greens or any other GiP-free vegetables from list in the tables

Fresh herbs – fresh mint leaves, lemon thyme or thyme leaves, coriander leaves, chives, dill, tarragon, basil leaves (use leftover herbs or dried herbs instead if you like)

Dressings

Thousand Island dressing, fat-free (or use any fat-free dressing you have)

Dairy chiller cabinet / chilled drinks
(you may have some left over)

Camembert cheese, small pack (try freezing what you don't need)

Hummus, half-fat, small tub

Ricotta cheese, small tub

Diet yoghurt, 3 (you may already have bought a multi-pack last trip)

Tomato juice, if you need / like it

Fresh / pre-cooked meat and fish / eggs

Cod fillet, fresh, weighing about 150 g (or you could buy frozen, see below)

Eggs, 3 (you may have some left over from last trip)

Cooked lean roast beef, 2 slices

Turkey breast, 1 skinless (if you buy a larger pack, freeze the rest raw; or cook for more than one day, chill in the fridge and then freeze leftovers)

For Sunday roast – choose one from:
> 3 slices of lean roast beef, OR 3 slices roast chicken breast, OR 1 roast chicken leg, OR chicken thigh or drumstick (skinless), OR 3 slices roast pork, OR 2 slices roast turkey, OR 2 slices lean roast lamb. Buy a little extra so you can use leftover meat for Monday's sandwich

Bread / bakery

(take out what you need and freeze the rest)

Pitta bread, small pack
Warburtons All In One Rolls

Canned vegetables / soups / fruit/ fish

Baby sweetcorn, 1 can
Soup, lentil, canned
Tomatoes: passata (sieved tomatoes) – 350 ml needed
Chilli beans, 1 can
Water chestnuts, 1 can
Sliced peaches, canned in juice
Tuna in brine, 1 can

Cereals

Muesli, small pack; and / or any 4-GiP breakfast cereal of your choice (see GiP tables). You may already have this
All Bran, small pack

Dried herbs, spices and flavourings

Dried herbs: herbes de Provence (or use herbs you already have)

Cajun spice

Paprika seasoning

Balsamic vinegar (optional – can use fat-free dressing already
   bought)

Chicken stock cube (or use vegetable stock from previous
   shopping trip)

Chilli sauce (optional)

Instant gravy powder (for Sunday roast)

Miscellaneous

Gherkins, small bottle (optional)

Oil, olive or rapeseed, small bottle

Olives, black or green, small bottle or pack

Sainsbury's Be Good to Yourself Chicken Tikka Masala and Rice
   (ready meal)

Snickers bar, fun-size, 1 (or buy standard size and cut into
   3 chunks, freeze the rest)

Yeast extract (e.g. Marmite), small jar

Frozen cod fillets, small pack (unless buying fresh)

Frozen vegetables

Broccoli

Also, if you prefer to buy frozen instead of fresh, check the
   vegetable section above and choose accordingly

New You Benefits

You will have started this during your two prep days. List your benefits here.

Your Fitness Burst Chart

For daily use. Use this chart to record how many of the 10-minute moderate-intensity activity sessions you're taking each day. Simply pencil in a tick every time, aiming for two ticks per day. If you manage more than 20 minutes a day, give yourself extra ticks.

Day	Fitness burst 1	Fitness burst 2
Tuesday		
Wednesday		
Thursday		
Friday		
Saturday		
Sunday		
Monday		
Tuesday		
Wednesday		
Thursday		

List Your Achievements

Here's your chance to write down all the wonderful things that you've managed to achieve each day of your 10-day plan. Remember, this can be simple things like choosing to go for a walk rather than sitting at your desk or in your armchair, or it can be something that you felt was more challenging, such as creating a meal from scratch and getting compliments for it. Whatever you choose to put on this list is for you, to motivate you and to congratulate yourself for everything you are achieving, no matter how small.

Rate Your Hunger

How hungry are you right now? Use these charts to help you get in tune with your appetite and fullness (satiety) cues (photocopy this page so that you can use the charts throughout the 10 days). Simply circle the appropriate number several times during one day or on several occasions on different days. As you become more aware of how hungry or full you are, you will be able to resist the temptation of eating something just because it is in front of you.

1 – Starving	1 – Starving
2 – Pretty hungry	2 – Pretty hungry
3 – Satisfied	3 – Satisfied
4 – Full	4 – Full
5 – Pigged out!	5 – Pigged out!
1 – Starving	1 – Starving
2 – Pretty hungry	2 – Pretty hungry
3 – Satisfied	3 – Satisfied
4 – Full	4 – Full
5 – Pigged out!	5 – Pigged out!

This exercise is described in more detail under Day 6 of your 10-day plan.

356 · PRACTICAL TOOLS

Your Goals?

Make these specific. For example, 'I choose to lose ½ an inch off my waist in 10 days' time.'

Practise the Plate

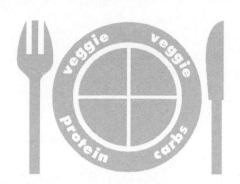

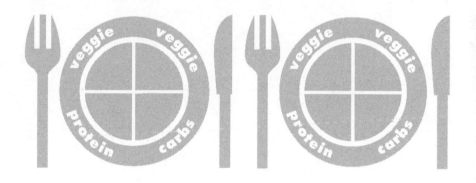

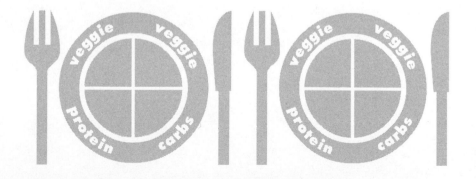

Rewards – List Them Here!

List Your Distractions

Trial and error! See what works for you.

Waist and Weight Progress Chart

Use this chart to record your progress. We suggest you make one recording before the 10 days, one on Celebration Friday, and one every two weeks after that. You should aim to lose around 0.5–1 kg (1–2 lb) each week.

Date	Waist measurement	Weight

Mood and Food Diary

Food fills a physical hole, not an emotional need. When you become more aware of the underlying feeling that is causing you to overeat, you are more able to make some changes. Fill in the daily food journal overleaf to highlight the emotional need that causes you to have a snack attack. Remind yourself, 'What would have to happen, that is within my control, for this need to be met in a healthy and functional way?' Before you seek solace in that 'naughty but nice food', ask yourself whether this is taking you nearer to the *new* you. If it isn't, choose again!

Recording what you eat will also help you to check if you are keeping to the GiP rules and, if not, what you might want to adjust next time. Photocopy the chart overleaf so you can analyse a few days.

Time	Food Eaten & Quantity	Fruit & Veg	GiPs

TOTAL GiPs FOR THE DAY

Week Number . . . .

Day/Date . . . .

Working/non-working day . . . .

Emotions, e.g. tired, hungry, feeling low	Comments

Ways You Can De-clutter

Notes

Notes

FURTHER SUPPORT & INFORMATION

Visit Az & Nina on www.giplan.com and www.thinkwelltobewell.com

www.giplan.com is a supportive site for anyone wanting to get into GI-eating by using the Gi Plan Diet, and contains motivational strategies. If you've already bought the book and need a quick inspirational 'top up', or some new menu ideas, this is worth a visit. For the uninitiated, www.giplan.com will simply whet your appetite.

www.thinkwelltobewell.com offers golden nuggets of information and inspires you to check and challenge your thinking, approach and attitudes to food choices and many aspects of life. It offers willpower boosters, slimming tips, and a host of information on diet and diabetes.

Workshops and programmes

Gi Plan Workshops will be held regularly throughout 2006, initially in an easily accessible location near to the M25/M4.

These are designed as highly practical, fun and inspirational days that will support you in achieving and/or sustaining your *new* you goals.

Email Az and Nina at: workshops@giplan.com

(Note, this address is for people interested in attending Gi Plan workshops only. We are unfortunately unable to provide personalised replies to GI queries.)

Art of intuition workshops
Learn to deal with hunger pangs and help yourself respond to stressful situations by using the creativity of your own 'gut feelings'.
www.artofintuition.co.uk

Get fit with Tonya

For tips on personal fitness, contact Antonia Parsons, RSA, who has helped with the physical activity tips in this book.
antonia@aj-associates.com

Books

The Gi Plan, Lose Weight Forever by Azmina Govindji and Nina Puddefoot. Published by Vermilion, 2004

Think Well To Be Well by Azmina Govindji and Nina Puddefoot. Published by Diabetes Research & Wellness Foundation, 2002

Other useful addresses and websites

Registered dietitians hold the only legally recognised graduate qualification in nutrition and dietetics. If you would like to visit a dietitian, send a stamped addressed envelope with your query to:

British Dietetic Association
5th Floor, Charles House, 148/9 Great Charles Street Queensway, Birmingham B3 3HT
Tel: 0121 200 8080

Diabetes Research & Wellness Foundation (DRWF)
The DRWF is a charity working to relieve the suffering of people with diabetes and related illnesses.
Diabetes Research and Wellness Foundation
Northney Marina, Hayling Island, Hants PO11 ONH
Tel: 023 9263 7808

Websites
The British Dietetic Association sites include:
www.bda.uk.com
www.weightwisebda.uk.com

For diabetes-specific sites, visit:
www.diabeteswellnessnet.org.uk
www.diabetes.org.uk

'Glycaemic Index – is it the right measure?', *The Nutrition Practitioner*, Summer 2005.
www.nutprac.com/5.html

Also try: www.govindjinutrition.com

INDEX